T0257116

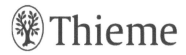

Plastic Surgery Oral Board Prep
Case Management Questions and Answers

Devra Becker, MD, FACS
Associate Professor of Plastic Surgery
Department of Plastic Surgery
University of Pittsburgh/UPMC
Pittsburgh, Pennsylvania

201 illustrations

Thieme
New York • Stuttgart • Delhi • Rio de Janeiro

Executive Editor: Stephan Konnry
Managing Editor: Elizabeth Palumbo
Director, Editorial Services: Mary Jo Casey
Production Editor: Sean Woznicki
International Production Director: Andreas Schabert
Editorial Director: Sue Hodgson
International Marketing Director: Fiona Henderson
International Sales Director: Louisa Turrell
Director of Institutional Sales: Adam Bernacki
Senior Vice President and Chief Operating Officer:
     Sarah Vanderbilt
President: Brian D. Scanlan

Library of Congress Cataloging-in-Publication Data

Names: Becker, Devra B., author.
Title: Plastic surgery oral board prep : case management
     questions and answers / Devra B. Becker.
Description: New York : Thieme, [2019] | Includes biblio
     graphical references. | Identifiers: LCCN
     2018025495 (print) | LCCN 2018026696 (ebook) |
     ISBN 9781626233522 (ebook) | ISBN 9781626233515
     (softcover)
Subjects: | MESH: Reconstructive Surgical Procedure—
     methods | Examination Questions
Classification: LCC RD118 (ebook) | LCC RD118 (print) |
     NLM WO 18.2 | DDC 617.9/52076—dc23
LC record available at https://lccn.loc.gov/2018025495

Important note: Medicine is an ever-changing science undergoing continual development. Research and clinical experience are continually expanding our knowledge, in particular our knowledge of proper treatment and drug therapy. Insofar as this book mentions any dosage or application, readers may rest assured that the authors, editors, and publishers have made every effort to ensure that such references are in accordance with **the state of knowledge at the time of production of the book.**

Nevertheless, this does not involve, imply, or express any guarantee or responsibility on the part of the publishers in respect to any dosage instructions and forms of applications stated in the book. **Every user is requested to examine carefully** the manufacturers' leaflets accompanying each drug and to check, if necessary in consultation with a physician or specialist, whether the dosage schedules mentioned therein or the contraindications stated by the manufacturers differ from the statements made in the present book. Such examination is particularly important with drugs that are either rarely used or have been newly released on the market. Every dosage schedule or every form of application used is entirely at the user's own risk and responsibility. The authors and publishers request every user to report to the publishers any discrepancies or inaccuracies noticed. If errors in this work are found after publication, errata will be posted at www.thieme.com on the product description page.

Some of the product names, patents, and registered designs referred to in this book are in fact registered trademarks or proprietary names even though specific reference to this fact is not always made in the text. Therefore, the appearance of a name without designation as proprietary is not to be construed as a representation by the publisher that it is in the public domain.

© 2019 Thieme Medical Publishers, Inc.

Thieme Publishers New York
333 Seventh Avenue, New York, NY 10001 USA
+1 800 782 3488, customerservice@thieme.com

Thieme Publishers Stuttgart
Rüdigerstrasse 14, 70469 Stuttgart, Germany
+49 [0]711 8931 421, customerservice@thieme.de

Thieme Publishers Delhi
A-12, Second Floor, Sector-2, Noida-201301
Uttar Pradesh, India
+91 120 45 566 00, customerservice@thieme.in

Thieme Publishers Rio de Janeiro, Thieme Publicações
     Ltda.
Edifício Rodolpho de Paoli, 25º andar
Av. Nilo Peçanha, 50 – Sala 2508,
Rio de Janeiro 20020-906 Brasil
+55 21 3172-2297 / +55 21 3172-1896
www.thiemerevinter.com.br

Cover design: Thieme Publishing Group
Typesetting by DiTech Process Solutions

Printed in The United States of America by   5 4 3 2 1
King Printing Co., Inc.

ISBN 978-1-62623-351-5

Also available as an e-book:
eISBN 978-1-62623-352-2

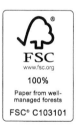

FSC
www.fsc.org
100%
Paper from well-
managed forests
FSC® C103101

For my parents, Judith and Stephen Beyer, and my sisters, Rebecca and Miriam, who help me fly and keep me grounded.

For Michal, Noa, Avi, and Sarah, who are my true legacy.

And קַל וָחוֹמֶר for my husband Lynton, who always makes me laugh and forgets nothing.

Contents

Contents

Foreword

There is no question that the pinnacle of formal categorical plastic surgery training, regardless of residency training program, is taking and passing the American Board of Plastic Surgery oral examination. This test essentially represents the culmination of decades' worth of education and dedication to learn skills, knowledge, craft, and art associated with the practice of plastic surgery. It also represents the last formal test in a long line of examinations that began likely in preschool (aside from maintenance of certification exams every 10 years). The amount of intense effort associated with studying for this exam translates into stress and pressure. In order to help mitigate that stress and pressure, examinee's pour their hearts and souls into preparation. That being said, when looking at the vast variety of resources available across the spectrum of plastic surgery to utilize to study for this exam, it is difficult to find one that solely focuses on oral exam preparation and concisely encapsulates practical information, is easy to read, digestible, and memorable. That is where Plastic Surgery Oral Board Prep comes in, authored by Dr. Devra Becker.

Dr. Becker has spent her career as an academic plastic surgeon. She has dedicated years specifically to training the next generation of plastic surgeons, and has done so at multiple academic medical centers, currently at the University of Pittsburgh Medical Center. She has also previously served as a Program Director for the residency training program at Case Western Reserve University School of Medicine in the Department of Plastic Surgery. Having served myself in a similar role at the University of Texas Southwestern Medical Center, I can assure you that is an incredibly labor-intensive, and yet phenomenally rewarding, position. In my mind, it represents significant altruism and dedication. Those same characteristics are evident when one reads this Plastic Surgery Oral Board Prep book given the amount of time, energy, and effort involved in undertaking such a project.

In this 22 chapter book, Dr. Becker does a brilliant job of trying to diffuse stress associated with taking the exam by condensing highpoint information into an easy-to-read format. Chapter one begins with an overview of the test, which is a natural starting point and gives backbone and context to the content that follows. The subsequent chapters cover topics such as preoperative assessment and perioperative management, postoperative events, cleft lip and palate, craniosynostosis syndromes, facial defect reconstruction, elective hand surgery, traumatic hand injuries, deep venous thrombosis prophylaxis, lower extremity reconstruction, , skin cancer, aesthetic surgery, breast reconstruction, elective breast surgery, back and trunk reconstruction, pressure ulcers, and others. There is even a chapter on ethical considerations, which is a critical addition considering this is an element of any training program and also the examination. All of these topics are relevant to the exam and are all organized in a standard question and answer format with well-illustrated graphics to help articulate content, and abbreviated bibliography to do a "deeper dive" if the reader would like additional source information.

One of the most helpful features of the book is that every chapter begins with "6 key points". These tables essentially summarize up front the chapter content to follow, and serve as a quick and dirty reference in case one wants to briefly review the take-home points associated with these chapters right before the exam.

At the end of the day, no matter how much preparation one does for the exam, there will always be a level of anxiety associated with it, as anyone knows who has taken the test. That being said, having a well written preparation book specifically tailored towards helping to prepare for this oral exam is a welcome, and valuable, addition to the bookshelves of anyone who is preparing to take the test.

Jeffrey Janis, MD, FACS
Professor of Plastic Surgery, Neurosurgery,
Neurology, and Surgery
Chief of Plastic Surgery, University Hospitals
Ohio State University
Wexner Medical Center

Preface

The plastic surgery oral board exam requires a unique skill set. Smart people, safe surgeons, and knowledgeable practitioners have all failed the oral board exam—not because they did not have the content knowledge, but because they did not synthesize the information appropriately.

The oral boards, to be sure, are daunting. But they are also the sine qua non of the plastic surgery training experience. Plastic surgeons traditionally have kept their oral board case books for decades—a singular feature of older plastic surgeons' offices is the stack of blue case books that they prepared for the exam.

Oral board review books historically have been focused on fact-based content rather than the holistic arc of a case, which is what informs the oral board exam. Coincident with my studying were the demands of setting up a practice. Decisions—large and small—about patient care were suddenly mine to make. These decisions, such as what medications to stop preoperatively or how soon and how often I would see a patient postoperatively, were not always readily available in my textbooks, and these questions began to influence how I studied for the exam.

Reflecting on my own experience, I realized to maximize success on the oral board exam, there needed to be a book that integrated core plastic surgery content with real-life application. Gathering together my notes, books, journal articles, and experience, I began to write a book of my own. As I developed my content, I discovered that my book would not only serve as preparation for the oral boards but also provide for the development of case management skills for future practice.

Information of representative cases is introduced in a way to encourage learning how to articulate the arc of a case. The questions and answers simulate a conversation, because that is what the exam is like. It is also like interactions with patients. Just as an examiner might say "the flap fails, what do you do now?," we say to patients "the flap might not take, and here is what we would do in that case." The answers are meant to be read aloud as part of the process of preparing for the oral boards. Projecting confidence and competence is important, and that can only be achieved by practicing answers aloud.

As I reflect back on my own studying, I realize that preparing for the exam honed my content knowledge and communication skills in a way no other experience has, and this knowledge and skill came in large part from working through cases in the way that this book presents them. Make it your own. Engage and learn.

1 General Approach to the Oral Board Examination

Abstract

This chapter will provide an overview of the examination process, and an algorithm for a general approach to cases. It will also provide strategies for addressing unfamiliar cases, and for redirecting one's answers when one makes an error during the examination.

Keywords: plastic surgery, plastic surgery oral board examination

Six Key Points

- Approach difficult and unfamiliar cases with a stepwise approach.
- Generate differential diagnoses.
- Always clearly state the diagnosis.
- Identify key points of diagnosis and management to communicate.
- Rehearse answers for when you get stuck.
- Plan and rehearse the flow of your answers for both straightforward and complex cases.

General Approach

The oral board examination is the final step in becoming a board-certified plastic surgeon. A knowledge base is essential, but a deficient knowledge base is not the only reason one may not be successful on the oral board examination. This book is designed to help you organize your knowledge to communicate it succinctly; it is a book about application of knowledge rather than mastery of knowledge. The first person is used in the answers, because in the oral board exam, as in practice, the answer to management questions is not what someone else would do, but what *you* would do.

Many plastic surgeons who are not successful in passing the oral board examination are not deficient in their knowledge. They struggle, however, with recalling the information in a practical way. It is a helpful exercise to distill how the questions on the oral board examination may be asked, and they are, in the most general terms, as follows: (1) *did you make the diagnosis correctly,* (2) *what are you going to do,* (3) *The algorithmic approach is useful for all to do it,* and (4) *what is your plan B when your plan A fails?*

Many textbooks focus on pictures, specific cases, and core knowledge. These are necessary but not sufficient components of your preparation. Part of your study strategy should be to be able to communicate your answers to the above four questions for any given diagnosis quickly and without relying on pictures. You should be able to take a cue word (e.g., aesthetic face or breast reconstruction) and discuss diagnostic considerations and treatment strategies, as well as management of complications.

This book is structured to help you do that.

Addressing Unfamiliar and Difficult Cases

The stepwise approach is useful for all cases, but its utility becomes clear in the unfamiliar case. It provides a general structure to organize your thought process, and helps ensure you will not overlook

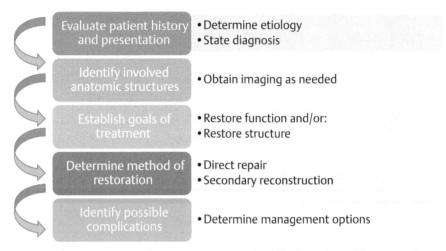

Evaluate patient history and presentation	• Determine etiology • State diagnosis
Identify involved anatomic structures	• Obtain imaging as needed
Establish goals of treatment	• Restore function and/or: • Restore structure
Determine method of restoration	• Direct repair • Secondary reconstruction
Identify possible complications	• Determine management options

Fig. 1.1 The stepwise approach to a case. These steps should be the anchors of diagnosis and decision-making.

significant findings. Most often, difficult cases are collections of smaller, manageable cases. **Fig. 1.1** provides a general approach to the difficult case.

Annotated Steps

1. The patient history and presentation is evaluated. A preliminary differential diagnosis is made. The etiology of the condition must be determined. The VINDICATE(M) mnemonic for the universal differential diagnosis can be helpful: Vascular, Infectious/Inflammatory, Neoplastic, Drugs/Degenerative, Iatrogenic/Idiopathic, Congenital, Autoimmune/Allergic, Trauma, Endocrine, (Metabolic).

2. If the etiology is unknown, one must determine the etiology of the condition. For example, suppose the case is a facial lesion in an adult. The etiology could be ectatic vessels (vascular), an injury (trauma), or it could be a squamous cell carcinoma or basal cell carcinoma (neoplastic.) You would determine the etiology by obtaining a tissue diagnosis. In the case of male

gynecomastia, etiologies could be endocrine, idiopathic, or drugs. One would work up the patient to exclude endocrine abnormalities prior to intervention. Once the etiology has been identified, it is important to state the diagnosis explicitly.

3. Once the etiology is identified, one determines the involved anatomic structures.

4. After the diagnosis has been made and the involved anatomic structures have been identified, one establishes the goals of treatment. Goals of treatment are, in general, to restore function and to restore structure. Once the functional goals are identified, they should be prioritized and triaged to likelihood of success. For example, an elderly patient with severe carpal tunnel syndrome manifested by night pain, constant numbness, and thenar atrophy may have identified goals of pain reduction and improvement in sensation, as well as improved muscle function. The goal of night pain reduction can be

achieved with a carpal tunnel release. The numbness may persist despite operative release. To restore function, one might consider a tendon transfer. In some cases, surgical intervention is not required to achieve the goals.

5. Once the functional goals are identified, one assesses whether there are structures that need to be restored. This is most apparent in trauma and tumor resection. Structural considerations are best approached with the *what is present and what is missing, what is missing and needs to be replaced, and what cannot be replaced?* model.

6. Finally, once one has an operative and nonoperative plan, one identifies potential complications.

Redirecting One's Answers

An important skill not only for the oral board examination, but also for general practice is being able to respond honestly and humbly while still projecting confidence and communicating your knowledge and content expertise. Planning how you will respond when you misspeak—and you will—helps make your answers concise, and helps avoid disorganized responses (**Fig. 1.2**).

Describing the Diagnosis

The ability to make a diagnosis is a key part of the oral board examination. Lead with your diagnosis. When describing radiographic imaging, the most succinct way of communicating the diagnosis is to use the formula as follows:

"*This* [AP/PA/LATERAL/OBLIQUE/CORONAL/AXIAL/SAGITTAL] *view of the* [BODY PART] *demonstrates* [DIAGNOSIS]."

Examples include the following:

- "This posteroanterior radiograph of the right hand demonstrates a boxer's fracture of the small finger metacarpal."

- "This coronal cut of a facial bone CT scan demonstrates a displaced right subcondylar mandibular fracture."

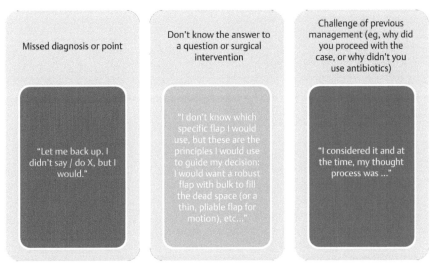

Missed diagnosis or point	Don't know the answer to a question or surgical intervention	Challenge of previous management (eg, why did you proceed with the case, or why didn't you use antibiotics)
"Let me back up. I didn't say / do X, but I would."	"I don't know which specific flap I would use, but these are the principles I would use to guide my decision: I would want a robust flap with bulk to fill the dead space (or a thin, pliable flap for motion), etc..."	"I considered it and at the time, my thought process was ..."

Fig. 1.2 Potential responses to missteps. A key to board preparation is rehearsing how you will handle situations in which you misspeak, do not know information, or are challenged about your management.

- "This oblique radiograph of the left wrist demonstrates scaphotrapezio-trapezoidal arthritis."

It is important to clearly state your diagnosis in the first few sentences, as thoroughly and as clearly as possible. Certain diagnoses seem obvious—*still say it*. "This is a stage 4 ischial pressure ulcer." "This is a Bennett fracture." If you need to clarify an eponymous diagnosis, you can say: "This is a Bennett fracture, an intra-articular fracture of the base of the thumb metacarpal bone that extends into the CMC joint."

A temptation is to state the diagnosis after you have described your supporting findings, as a conclusion rather than as an opening statement. "I'm looking at a radiograph of the hand; the soft tissues look intact with some swelling, the phalanges look intact, there are no fractures of the small, ring, middle, or index fingers. There is a fracture of the base of the thumb metacarpal." This strategy wastes time. Rather, the first few sentences should state your conclusion, followed by your supporting evidence: "This radiograph of the hand demonstrates a Bennett fracture. I do not see other fractures in the phalanges or metacarpals, or evidence of soft-tissue injury." This communicates that you have made the diagnosis, but have also assessed for other injury in a clear and straightforward way.

Assessing the Pace of a Case

There is a short amount of time for each case, but each case may vary in complexity. In some cases, making the diagnosis is the hardest part of the case, and operative decision-making is standard and flows from the diagnosis—for example, a Skier's thumb. In other cases, the diagnosis is given to you (acquired absence of the breast with radiation therapy for breast cancer) and the hardest part is getting through all of the material—deciding on the procedure, drawing markings, and perioperative care and management of complications and suboptimal results. In each case, make a list of highlights for each stage of care—diagnosis, operative intervention, postoperative care, and management of complications—to be discussed. This will help keep you on pace.

Interpreting Radiographs By Teresa Chapman, MD

Proper interpretation of any diagnostic study, including radiographs, begins with having a systematic method for assessing the images. Develop a system, and stick with it. Here is a simple approach that you might find useful.

1. Bone mineralization

This takes experience, to calibrate your eyes for the spectrum of normal. Essentially, though, your goal is to determine if the bones are "white" (dense) enough. When bones begin to demineralize, which puts them at risk for fracture, they begin to look less white, the bony trabeculae begin to stand out, and the cortices of long bones (particularly in the hands and feet) begin to thin.

2. Soft tissues

Step back and ignore the bones for a moment to assess the soft tissues. The soft tissues may direct your eyes to a relevant bone finding. Is there superficial density reflecting edema infiltrating the subcutaneous fat? Are the deeper soft tissues or fad pads displaced away from the bone? Symmetry is your friend. If you have the chance to compare with the contralateral side, that can be very helpful. Look for soft-tissue mineralization and foreign bodies as well as for soft-tissue edema.

3. Focal bone findings

Fractures are sharply marginated lucencies. A common pitfall in radiograph interpretation is mistaking a vascular channel through bone (a normal finding) for a fracture. Vascular channels have smooth margins, uniform width, and usually a straight or curved path. Osteochondral defects are semilunar lucencies at the articular surfaces of certain bones, like femoral condyles, talar dome, and capitellum. Bone tumors may appear as lucencies or as sclerotic (dense) abnormalities, and the shape and definition of a bone tumor's margins help a radiologist in determining if it is aggressive or benign.

4. Joint spaces

Again, symmetry is your friend. Individuals have different joint space widths, and so you must rely on consistency within a single patient. Look for joint space narrowing as an indication of arthritis, and look for joint space widening as an indicator of effusion or traumatic subluxation.

5. Completion of film interrogation

Always remember to look at every single bone on every single view. It is standard to assess hands and feet using three radiographic projections (anteroposterior or posteroanterior, oblique, and lateral). Phalangeal fractures are easy to miss if you do not look for them. Finally, always remind yourself to study the corners of the images. The important findings are not always in the center of the image.

2 Preoperative Assessment and Perioperative Management

Abstract

This chapter will provide an overview of preoperative assessment as it relates to plastic surgery. It will include medication management and will review perioperative antibiotic management. The reader will be able to prepare management plans for different scenarios.

Keywords: preoperative assessment, perioperative management, DVT, antibiotic prophylaxis, SCIP

Six Key Points

- The Surgical Care Improvement Project (SCIP) defines postoperative events and makes recommendations on perioperative management.
- Superficial plastic surgery cases are low risk.
- Patients with cardiac stents should remain on anticoagulation.
- Smoking increases complications fivefold.
- Patients should stop smoking 8 weeks prior to elective surgery.
- Assess the risk of obstructive sleep apnea.

Overview

While the preoperative workup can be tailored to a specific problem, there are general principles of perioperative management that are useful for any case. The Surgical Care Improvement Project (SCIP) was created in 2003 as an initiative of the Centers for Disease Control and Prevention (CDC) and Centers for Medicare & Medicaid Services (CMS), and has a defined goal to reduce surgical morbidity and vmortality. It has defined postoperative events and makes recommendations on perioperative management.

Questions

Case 1

Preoperative Assessment

1. What is considered low-risk surgery?
Superficial plastic surgery cases and general breast surgery are considered low-risk surgeries. Low-risk surgery can become moderate risk surgery if general anesthesia is required.

2. What are the revised cardiac risk indicators?
Invasive surgery, ischemic heart disease, heart failure, cerebrovascular accident (CVA), creatinine greater than 2.0, and diabetes mellitus requiring insulin.

3. Your patient was found to have a cardiac condition and had stents placed. Under what conditions do you proceed with surgical intervention?
If a patient has had a previous balloon angioplasty over 14 days ago, one can proceed with surgery if the patient continues aspirin. If the patient has a bare-metal stent, and it has been more than 6 weeks (ideally 3 months), the patient can be taken to surgery with aspirin. If the patient has had a drug-eluting stent, nonurgent

surgery should be postponed until after a year, and then surgery can proceed if the patient continues aspirin.

Medication Management

1. Your patient wants to know which medications he can take before surgery (Table 2.1). What do you tell him?
Some medications can be taken up to and including the day of surgery, some should be taken until surgery but not taken on the day of surgery, and some should be stopped prior to surgery. These are summarized in **Table 2.1**.

Pulmonary

1. Your patient is a smoker. What sorts of perioperative pulmonary risks are associated with smoking?
All complications (major and minor) related to smoking are increased almost fivefold when compared with never smokers. Past smokers are also at increased risk.[1]

2. How long should a patient have quit smoking prior to surgery?
Ideally, a patient should have quit smoking for at least 8 weeks prior to elective surgery.[2]

3. How do you verify the patient has quit smoking prior to surgery?
One always has discussion with patients regarding smoking prior to surgery. Identification and verification of smoking cessation is a two-pronged approach: direct discussion with the patient and a serum cotinine test.
RATIONALE: A serum cotinine test can be ordered either qualitatively or quantitatively. The quantitative test will help distinguish between an active tobacco user and one who has recently quit; it takes approximately 2 weeks for serum cotinine to return to normal.

Table 2.1 Perioperative management of medications

Category	Medication	Indication	Until surgery	Day of surgery
Heart failure	Beta blockers		Yes	Yes
	ACE/ARB		Yes	No
	Diuretics		Yes	No
	Hydralazine/nitrates			
Anticoagulation	Aspirin	Primary prevention of CAD/stroke	Yes	Yes
		Stents	Yes	Yes
	Clopidogrel		Yes	Yes
	Prasugrel		Yes	Yes
	Piclodipine		Yes	Yes
Oncologic	Tamoxifen		Stop 5 d before	No
	Aromatase inhibitors		Yes	Yes
Diabetes	Insulin (long acting)		Yes	No
	Insulin (short acting)		Yes	No
Psychiatric	MAOI		Stop 2 wk before	No

Abbreviations: ACE, angiotensin-converting enzyme; ARB, angiotensin receptor blocker; CAD, coronary artery disease; MAOI, monoamine oxidase inhibitor.

Active smokers have serum cotinine greater than 14 ng/mL, recent smokers have levels of 0.5 to 13.9 ng/mL, and unexposed people have serum cotinine levels less than 0.05 ng/mL.[3]

4. How do you assess the risk of obstructive sleep apnea (OSA) in a patient?

I assess the risk of OSA with the STOP-Bang score.

RATIONALE: The STOP-Bang score, published in 2008 and 2012,[4,5] is used to assess risk of OSA. It assigns 1 point for each answer of yes to the following screening questions:

- Do you Snore?
- Are you Tired during the day?
- Witnessed Obstruction when asleep?
- High blood Pressure?
- BMI greater than 35 kg/m²?
- Age older than 50 years?
- Neck size greater than 17 inches in males and greater than 16 inches in females?
- And male Gender?

A score of 0 to 2 is low risk, 3 to 4 is intermediate risk, and greater than 5 is high risk. A score of 6 or higher is most predictive. The STOP-Bang questionnaire has been validated in obese and morbidly obese patients.[6]

Case 2

Perioperative Management

1. When do you start and stop perioperative antibiotics?

Antibiotics are given within one hour of surgery and are discontinued within 48 hours after surgery.

RATIONALE: The SCIP measures include postoperative infection as a surgical complication. The recommendations are to receive IV antibiotics within 1 hour of incision, and antibiotics given more than 2 hours before incision or after incision are both associated with greater rates of wound infection.[7] The criteria for antibiotic prophylaxis are that the antibiotic should be safe, cost-effective, and broad spectrum. Prophylactic antibiotics should be discontinued within 48 hours of surgical end time.

There is some controversy regarding postoperative use of antibiotics. The American Society of Plastic Surgeons notes that there are no good recommendations regarding antibiotics with the use of drains. Some studies have shown that when postoperative antibiotics are continued longer than recommended, antibiotic resistance is more prevalent when infection does occur.

2. What is your intraoperative and postoperative deep vein thrombosis (DVT) prophylaxis protocol?

DVT prophylaxis begins with assessment of risk, which is performed by calculating the Caprini score (**Fig. 2.1**).

RATIONALE: The Caprini score is a point system in which patient-specific factors such as obesity, age, history, and type and length of surgery are considered and assigned points. A score of 0 to 1 is low risk (2% incidence of DVT), 2 is moderate risk (10–20% incidence), 3 to 4 is high risk (20–40% incidence), and 5 is highest risk (40–80%). Treatment for each score is presented in **Table 2.2**.

Early ambulation is a mainstay of prevention for all plastic surgery patients and is undertaken as soon as it is safe to do so surgically. In addition, for body contouring patients, enoxaparin is given for a 7- to 10-day postoperative course.

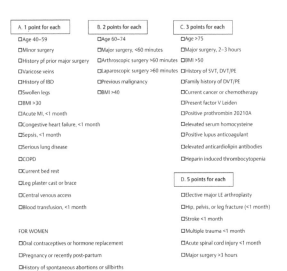

A. 1 point for each	B. 2 points for each	C. 3 points for each
☐Age 40–59	☐Age 60–74	☐Age >75
☐Minor surgery	☐Major surgery, <60 minutes	☐Major surgery, 2–3 hours
☐History pf prior major surgery	☐Arthroscopic surgery >60 minutes	☐BMI >50
☐Varicose veins	☐Laparoscopic surgery >60 minutes	☐History of SVT, DVT/PE
☐History of IBD	☐Previous malignancy	☐Family history of DVT/PE
☐Swollen legs	☐BMI >40	☐Current cancer or chemotherapy
☐BMI >30		☐Present factor V Leiden
☐Acute MI, <1 month		☐Positive prothrombin 20210A
☐Congestive heart failure, <1 month		☐elevated serum homocysteine
☐Sepsis, <1 month		☐Positive lupus anticoagulant
☐Serious lung disease		☐elevated anticardiolipin antibodies
☐COPD		☐Heparin induced thrombocytopenia
☐Current bed rest		
☐Leg plaster cast or brace		**D. 5 points for each**
☐Central venous access		☐Elective major LE arthroplasty
☐Blood transfusion, <1 month		☐Hip, pelvis, or leg fracture (<1 month)
		☐Stroke <1 month
FOR WOMEN		☐Multiple trauma <1 month
☐Oral contraceptives or hormone replacement		☐Acute spinal cord injury <1 month
☐Pregnancy or recently post-partum		☐Major surgery >3 hours
☐History of spontaneous abortions or sillbirths		

Fig. 2.1 Caprini score. The Caprini score is a validated method of predicting deep vein thrombosis/pulmonary embolism risk, and proposes intervention based on measured risk. (Adapted from Caprini JA. Risk assessment as a guide to thrombosis prophylaxis. Curr Opin Pulm Med 2010;16(5):448–452.)

Table 2.2 Caprini score risk stratification and recommendations

Caprini score	Risk	Prophylaxis
0–1	Low (2%)	Early ambulation
2	Moderate (10–20%)	Mechanical prophylaxis (sequential compression device) OR chemoprophylaxis (heparin 5,000 units SQ twice daily)
3–4	High (20–40%)	Chemoprophylaxis (heparin or enoxaparin weight-based and renally based dosing) ± mechanical prophylaxis
≥5	Highest (40–80%)	Chemoprophylaxis (Lovenox is preferred, heparin preferred with epidurals) AND mechanical prophylaxis

Abbreviation: SQ, subcutaneous.

References

1. Bluman LG, Mosca L, Newman N, Simon DG. Preoperative smoking habits and postoperative pulmonary complications. Chest 1998;113(4):883–889
2. Smetana GW. Preoperative pulmonary evaluation. N Engl J Med 1999;340(12):937–944
3. Benowitz NL, Schultz KE, Haller CA, Wu AH, Dains KM, Jacob P III. Prevalence of smoking assessed biochemically in an urban public hospital: a rationale for routine cotinine screening. Am J Epidemiol 2009;170(7):885–891
4. Chung F, Yegneswaran B, Liao P, et al. STOP questionnaire: a tool to screen patients for obstructive sleep apnea. Anesthesiology 2008;108(5): 812–821
5. Chung F, Subramanyam R, Liao P, Sasaki E, Shapiro C, Sun Y. High STOP-Bang score indicates a high probability of obstructive sleep apnoea. Br J Anaesth 2012;108(5):768–775
6. Ching F, Ynag Y, Liao P. Predictive performance of the STOP-Bang score for identifying obstructive sleep apnea in obese patients. Obes Surg 2013;23(12):2050–2057
7. Gyssens IC. Preventing postoperative infections: current treatment recommendations. Drugs 1999;57(2):175–185

3 Venous Thromboembolism Prophylaxis

Abstract

This chapter will provide current best practices of venous thromboembolism (VTE) prophylaxis. VTE is a disease process that includes deep venous thrombosis (DVT) and pulmonary embolism (PE). The reader will be able to integrate recommendations from multiple sources and justify given prophylaxis protocols.

Keywords: venous thromboembolism, deep venous thrombosis, pulmonary embolus, Caprini score

Six Key Points

- Risk stratification is based on the Caprini score.
- Venous thromboembolism prophylaxis should continue for 1 month after surgery.
- Risks factors include surgery, cancer, immobility, prior history, age, and obesity.
- A patient with a postoperative deep venous thrombosis (DVT) should remain anticoagulated for 6 months.
- A patient with a postoperative DVT should get a hypercoagulable workup.
- Workup should be 6 months after event.

Questions

1. How do you risk stratify patients for venous thromboembolism (VTE)?

Different methods are used for risk stratification for VTE. A common method, and one used in the plastic surgery literature reviewing VTE risk after surgery, is the Caprini score.[1,2]

2. Your patient had a prior VTE. How should the patient be risk stratified?

According to the American College of Chest Physicians (ACCP) guidelines, the suggested risk stratification for VTE is high risk with a VTE less than 3 months prior or with severe thrombophilia, such as antiphospholipid antibodies; moderate risk includes patients who have had a VTE within 3 to 12 months and nonsevere thrombophilia, such as a heterozygous factor V mutation, recurrent VTE, or active cancer; and low risk is a prior VTE greater than 2 months ago and no other risk factors.

3. What are known risk factors for VTE?

Known risk factors for VTE are surgery, cancer, immobilization, prior history, age, and obesity.[3] Virchow's triad includes venous stasis, vascular injury, and/or hypercoagulability. Surgery itself causes venous stasis, because of vasodilation from general anesthesia and after intravenous saline infusion.[4] Vascular injury can occur during surgery, and other risk factors are documented in the Caprini score.

4. How long should patients be on postoperative VTE prophylaxis?

For patients undergoing major abdominal surgery, a Cochrane review[5] indicated that prophylaxis should be given for 1 month after surgery. The review was based on three randomized controlled trials in manuscript form, and one randomized controlled trial in abstract form. They noted that a benefit of fewer symptomatic VTE was found in prolonged prophylactic therapy, without an increase in the risk of bleeding.

Postoperative enoxaparin has been shown to be beneficial in high-risk plastic surgery patients.[6]

5. Your patient is postoperative day (POD) 6 after body contouring for massive weight loss and call the office with reports of right calf tenderness. He reports he was working out the day prior and thinks he may have strained his calf muscle, and would like to take a muscle relaxant with his pain medication. What do you do?

This patient should go to the emergency room to rule out a DVT, which can present as calf tenderness. Workup should include a Doppler ultrasound. A high-sensitivity D dimer is often used in the workup of DVT, but can be elevated after recent surgery.

6. What sequelae can patients get after DVT?

The most feared event after a DVT is a pulmonary embolus (PE), which has a fatality risk. Even without PE, patients can get phlegmasia alba dolens (white swollen leg), phlegmasia cerulea dolens (blue swollen leg), venous gangrene, and postthrombotic syndrome, which is characterized by pain and leg swelling.[7]

7. How long should patients be on anticoagulation therapy after a DVT?

Patients should be on anticoagulation for at least 3 months after a DVT, and up to 6 to 12 months depending on risk factors (**Fig. 3.1**).

8. Should patients have a workup for a hypercoagulable state after a DVT?

Patients with a DVT after surgery should have a workup, especially if it was unexpected. Because the presence of a thrombus and the use of anticoagulation can interfere with the workup, it is best to perform the workup 6 months after the event, after treatment has been completed.

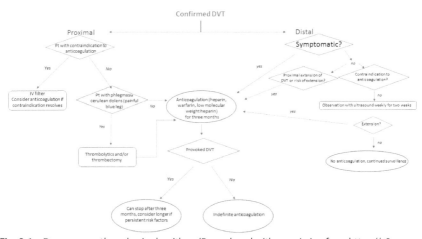

Fig. 3.1 Deep venous thrombosis algorithm. (Reproduced with permission from https://s0www.utdlab.com/contents/image?imageKey=PULM%2F97117.)

References

1. Pannucci CJ, Bailey SH, Dreszer G, et al. Validation of the Caprini risk assessment model in plastic and reconstructive surgery patients. J Am Coll Surg 2011;212(1):105–112
2. Pannucci CJ, Barta RJ, Portschy PR, et al. Assessment of postoperative venous thromboembolism risk in plastic surgery patients using the 2005 and 2010 Caprini Risk score. Plast Reconstr Surg 2012;130(2):343–353
3. Kahn SR, Morrison DR, Cohen JM, et al. Interventions for implementation of thromboprophylaxis in hospitalized medical and surgical patients at risk for venous thromboembolism. Cochrane Database Syst Rev 2013;16(7):CD008201
4. Coleridge-Smith PD, Hasty JH, Scurr JH. Venous stasis and vein lumen changes during surgery. Br J Surg 1990;77(9):1055–1059
5. Rasmussen MS, Jørgensen LN, Wille-Jørgensen P. Prolonged thromboprophylaxis with low molecular weight heparin for abdominal or pelvic surgery. Cochrane Database Syst Rev 2009;29(1):CD004318
6. Pannucci CJ, Dreszer G, Wachtman CF, et al. Postoperative enoxaparin prevents symptomatic venous thromboembolism in high-risk plastic surgery patients. Plast Reconstr Surg 2011;128(5):1093–1103
7. Bahl V, Hu HM, Henke PK, Wakefield TW, Campbell DA Jr, Caprini JA. A validation study of a retrospective venous thromboembolism risk scoring method. Ann Surg 2010;251(2):344–350

4 Postoperative Events: Fat Embolism and Compartment Syndrome

Abstract

This chapter will provide an overview of common life- and limb-threatening events fat embolus and compartment syndrome. The reader will be able to diagnose these conditions through their hallmark presentations, and demonstrate application of algorithms for treatment.

Keywords: fat embolus, compartment syndrome, compartment pressures

Six Key Points

- Fat embolism presents as hypoxemia, petechial rash, and mental status changes.
- Fat embolism is a clinical diagnosis.
- Treatment for fat embolism is supportive.
- Compartment syndrome presents with the five 'Ps."
- Compartment syndrome is a clinical diagnosis, although compartment pressures of > 30mmHg are an indication to perform a fasciotomy
- Treatment of compartment syndrome is surgical, and post-operative care includes frequent neurovascular assessments

Questions

Case 1

A woman calls 4 days after an abdominoplasty and liposuction and reports that she has shortness of breath.

1. What do you do?

She should be evaluated in clinic, and it should include vital signs, examination of the surgical site, evaluation of the lower extremities, and cardiac and pulmonary evaluation, and general skin assessment. Leg swelling must be evaluated to rule out a deep venous thrombosis (DVT), and if leg swelling is the only symptom, imaging should include a duplex ultrasound to rule out a DVT. If a patient has pulmonary symptoms, such as shortness of breath, or has a low-grade fever, a spiral CT/pulmonary embolism (PE) protocol should be considered.

RATIONALE: A study using national databases to evaluate postoperative complications found that DVT/PE occurred at a rate of 0.1 or 0.3% (depending on the database) when performed alone, and 0.4 or 0.27% when combined with another procedure.[1]

2. The patient comes to the clinic, and has a rash. What do you do?

A petechial rash is concerning for fat embolism syndrome, which can occur after liposuction. Initial diagnostic imaging should include chest imaging with a chest X-ray and a CT.

RATIONALE: The signs and symptoms of the syndrome usually present between 24 and 72 hours after the inciting event (surgery), and are most commonly seen on the neck and axillae. There are three features of fat embolism: hypoxemia, petechial rash, and mental status changes. Pulmonary symptoms usually occur early in the time course of the syndrome. The petechial rash is typically the last symptom to present, and present in approximately one-third of cases.[2]

While there are characteristic features of fat embolism syndrome, it is a clinical diagnosis. It is considered a diagnosis of exclusion as the features of the syndrome are nonspecific. The differential diagnosis should exclude other etiologies of emboli, such as thrombus. Of the conditions included in the differential diagnosis, the one that bears the most similarity to fat embolism syndrome is silicone embolism syndrome, which occurs after silicone has been injected. While treatment for silicone embolism syndrome is supportive as well, the prognosis in patients who have neurological symptoms with silicone embolism syndrome is worse.

3. You have diagnosed fat embolism syndrome. What do you do now?
Treatment is supportive. The patient should be admitted to the hospital, and given supplemental oxygen and fluid resuscitation as needed. If escalated respiratory support is needed, such as mechanical ventilation, it should be instituted.
RATIONALE: There is no single therapeutic intervention for fat embolism syndrome. In most cases, patients with fat embolism syndrome recover with supportive care, and recovery can occur as quickly as several days.

Case 2

You are managing a 68-year-old male patient in-house for a scalp rotation flap after resection of a scalp squamous cell carcinoma; he is on warfarin and his most recent international normalized ratio (INR) was 2.8. Nursing calls to inform you that he has fallen, and his forearm appears swollen.

1. What do you do?
The primary differential diagnoses are hematoma, generalized swelling, orthopaedic trauma/broken bones, or compartment syndrome.

Initial assessment includes thorough history of the events surrounding the fall, and whether it was associated with a loss of consciousness, to rule out underlying cerebral or cardiac events. Assuming there is no reason to suspect cerebral events such as stroke as a causative factor or brain injury as a resultant factor, or cardiac events, the time course of the swelling is assessed. A full physical examination is conducted and includes examination and assessment for a localized fluid collection, assessment of movement (flexion and extension), a full nerve examination, and pulse assessment.

2. What else do you do?
A radiograph should be taken to rule out underlying fracture, but a concern in a swollen, tense arm after a fall in an anticoagulated patient is compartment syndrome.
RATIONALE: The clinical signs of compartment syndrome are pain, pallor, paresthesias, pulselessness, and poikilothermia. Pulselessness is often a late finding (**Fig. 4.1**). Compartment pressures should be measured, and there are multiple ways to measure compartment pressure.
RATIONALE:
- Warfarin Available Kits (e.g., Stryker): The Stryker monitor is a handheld device that uses readily available equipment. It allows for continuous monitoring and requires minimal setup.
- Whitesides' Method: Whitesides and Heckman[3] described a method of measuring tissue pressures that utilizes a 20-mL syringe, IV extension tubing, a hypodermic needle, and a manometer (**Fig. 4.2**). While this requires setup, it uses equipment that is readily available in a hospital setup.
- Matsen's Continuous Infusion: Matsen described a technique of measuring compartment pressures with a pressure transducer and monitor, and an infusion pump (**Fig. 4.3**).[4] Though

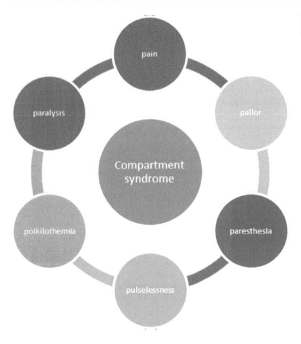

Fig. 4.1 Signs and symptoms of compartment syndrome.

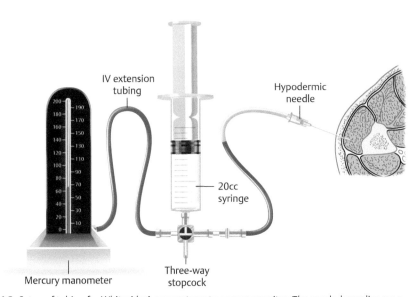

Fig. 4.2 Setup of tubing for Whitesides' compartment pressure monitor. The needed supplies are a mercury manometer, IV extension tubing, a three-way stopcock, a hypodermic needle, and a 20-mL syringe. Note the saline meniscus must be level with the needle for an accurate reading. (Adapted from Whitesides TE, Heckman MM. Acute compartment syndrome: update on diagnosis and treatment. J Am Acad Orthop Surg 1996;4(4):209–218)

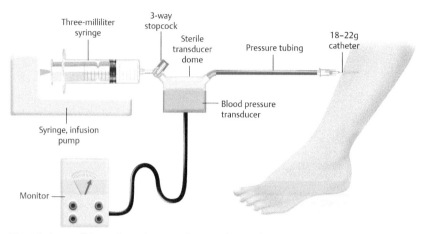

Fig. 4.3 Setup of Matsen's continuous infusion technique for monitoring compartment pressures. As originally described, it requires a 3-mL syringe (S), infusion pump (I), three-way stopcock (K), sterile transducer dome (D) with a blood pressure transducer (T), pressure tubing (P), 18- to 22-G catheter (C), and monitor (M). (Adapted from Matsen FA III, Winquist RA, Krugmire RB Jr. Diagnosis and management of compartmental syndromes. J Bone Joint Surg Am 1980;62(2):286–291)

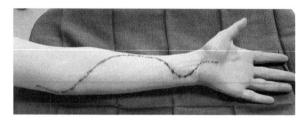

Fig. 4.4 Fasciotomy incisions in the forearm. A single incision can release all of the forearm compartments and the carpal tunnel. A second incision can be performed over the radial wad, if needed.

equipment is not always readily available, continuous monitoring of tissue pressure can occur for 3 days. While advocated for equivocal cases, the authors of the original study noted that individuals varied in their tolerance of increased compartmental pressures, and emphasized the clinical nature of the diagnosis.

- Wick Catheter Technique: Described in the late 1960s, the wick catheter technique uses polyglycolic acid suture threaded through an epidural catheter filled with heparinized saline and attached to a manometer.[5] The theoretical advantage of the wick is that it does not require infusion of fluid, and thus the pressure measured is at equilibrium.

In general, compartment pressures greater than 30 mm Hg are an indication to perform a fasciotomy and are consistent with a diagnosis of compartment syndrome.

3. How do you proceed?

If there is a clinical suspicion of compartment syndrome, an emergent fasciotomy is performed in the operating room. The carpal tunnel is released, and a curvilinear incision is made directed toward Guyon's canal, making a gentle sine wave radially centrally in the forearm, and then curving ulnarly to the cubital tunnel (**Fig. 4.4**).

Once the incisions are made, the fascia is released with scissors. The color and general appearance of the muscle are noted, and hematoma is evacuated as needed. Necrotic tissue can be debrided. The incisions can be closed loosely or can be left open.

4. What is your postoperative protocol?

Postoperatively, loose dressings are placed on the arm, and it is important that no dressings be constrictive. Daily examinations are performed that include, as preoperatively, a thorough neurovascular assessment. Occupational therapy is started for range of motion.

References

1. Alderman AK, Collins ED, Streu R, etal. Benchmarking outcomes in plastic surgery: national complication rates for abdominoplasty and breast augmentation. Plast Reconstr Surg 2009;124(6):2127–2133

2. Weinhouse GL. Fat embolism syndrome. In: Parsons PE, ed. Literature Review Current through 1/2017, Last Updated 1/17/2017. Waltham, MA: UpToDate, Inc

3. Whitesides TE, Heckman MM. Acute compartment syndrome: update on diagnosis and treatment. J Am Acad Orthop Surg 1996;4(4):209–218

4. Matsen FA III, Winquist RA, Krugmire RB Jr. Diagnosis and management of compartmental syndromes. J Bone Joint Surg Am 1980;62(2):286–291

5. Mubarak SJ, Hargens AR, Owen CA, Garetto LP, Akeson WH. The wick catheter technique for measurement of intramuscular pressure. A new research and clinical tool. J Bone Joint Surg Am 1976;58(7):1016–1020

5 Free Flap Failure

Abstract

This chapter will review postoperative monitoring of the free flap patient and management of free flap failure. The reader will be able to discriminate between arterial and venous free flap failure, and explain operative and nonoperative interventions for free flap failure.

Keywords: free flap failure, arterial compromise, venous compromise, free flap salvage, free flap monitoring

Six Key Points

- Postoperative monitoring should include conventional methods of color, turgor, and warmth.
- Signs of failure are a purple flap or a white flap.
- Conservative measures first.
- Operative intervention to rule out extrinsic causes or intrinsic causes.
- Heparinize ± thrombectomy for early clot, heparin/thrombectomy/thrombolytics for established clot.
- Salvage options include second free flap, local flap, or delayed flap.

Overview

All free flaps—whether in breast reconstruction, lower extremity reconstruction, or other reconstruction—have the potential for failure. The key is being able to identify *cause* quickly and have a *management plan*. A systematic approach will be outlined here.

Questions

1. What is your postoperative monitoring protocol?

Flap checks should occur at prescribed intervals, such as every hour for 24 hours, then every 2 hours after that. Flap checks should include bedside assessment of color, temperature, turgor, capillary refill, and Doppler monitoring. Flap checks also include assessment of the signal from an implantable Doppler.

Color is assessed by visual inspection, and a picture of the flap immediately after surgery can be hung at the bedside to allow comparison. The temperature can be measured from a skin paddle, and in some cases of buried flaps, a component may be externalized to allow monitoring. Temperature can be measured from palpation on physical examination, probes, and temperature tape. Capillary refill is described as either normal, brisk, or slow, and Doppler monitoring should be performed at the same spot, marked with a stitch (**Fig. 5.1**).

Patients should also receive aspirin every day, and subcutaneous heparin 5,000 units twice daily.

RATIONALE: Adjunctive techniques include implantable Doppler systems, color duplex sonography, near-infrared spectroscopy, laser Doppler flowmetry (LDF), and microdialysis. Though expensive, adjunctive techniques identify free flap compromise earlier than conventional methods alone, and a review suggested that despite limitations of studies comparing methods, some adjunctive methods

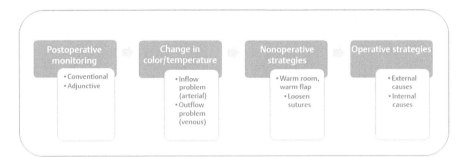

Fig. 5.1 Postoperative monitoring and intervention algorithm of free flaps.

should be used. Implantable Doppler systems have the advantage of being the least expensive of these, and are straightforward, which makes them useful for novices. Near-infrared spectroscopy was thought to be reliable with a 100% positive and negative predictive value, and is noninvasive, and was thought to be promising as an "ideal monitoring system."[1]

2. What are an implantable Doppler, color duplex sonography, near-infrared spectroscopy, LDF, and microdialysis?

- Implantable Doppler: An implantable Doppler (or internal Doppler) is a device that wraps around a microvascular anastomosis, typically the vein because the vein is considered more rapid and accurate.[2] Implantable Doppler systems, though accurate, can fail, and should not be the sole source of assessment of a flap.
- Color Duplex Sonography: Color duplex sonography is a noninvasive monitoring technique that evaluates blood flow velocity and direction. It is not a continuous monitoring system, and provides information only at the time of analysis. Though accurate and precise, it requires an ultrasound technician and intimate knowledge of the flap anatomy, which may mean that

both the microsurgeon and the ultrasonographer must be present for the evaluation. It is most often used for buried flaps.
- Near-Infrared Spectroscopy: Near-infrared spectroscopy is a noninvasive technique that uses optical spectroscopy to measure oxygenated and deoxygenated hemoglobin through absorption spectra. The tissue penetration of the light has been reported to be up to 20 mm, and can be used for most flaps.[3]
- LDF is a noninvasive technique that uses coherent, collimated, monochromatic laser light transmitted through fiberoptic cables. The probe collects backscattered light, which fluctuates in intensity, and creates a function of low. The limitations of LDF are that one must follow trends rather than absolute readings, and it is very prone to artifacts, including positioning.
- Microdialysis is an invasive technique in which a double-lumen catheter is placed in the tissues and dialysate is infused into the tissues; as it equilibrates with the extracellular matrix, it is sampled in microvials and analyzed for glucose, lactate, pyruvate, and glycerol. In arterial compromise, the glucose levels decrease and lactate:

pyruvate ratio increases. Glycerol is a nonspecific sign of cell membrane damage and is seen in both arterial and venous compromise. While this has the advantage of identifying compromise before clinical signs appear, it only measures the tissue physiology at the sampling site.[4]

3. An implantable Doppler is not available. What do you do?

If an implantable Doppler is not available, conventional methods are used to evaluate the flap at the same intervals as above.

4. How long do you monitor your free flaps?

At least 3 days for breast free flaps, and at least 5 days for head and neck free flaps.

RATIONALE: Studies have shown that most breast complications occur within 48 hours, but most head and neck complications occur within 5 days. Therefore, one has to monitor head and neck reconstructions longer.[5] Ninety percent of arterial thromboses occur within the first 24 hours.

5. A nurse calls to tell you that the flap looks white and cool. What do you do?

A pale and cool flap has an inflow (arterial) problem, and arterial thrombus must be ruled out. One must evaluate the flap, and ensure that the environment is appropriate, including a warm room, warm blankets around the flap, and sufficient resuscitation of the patient. The flap should be evaluated for bleeding, and a pinprick test should elicit bleeding; however, the likely cause of a pale flap is a thrombus, and as nonoperative strategies are being undertaken, operative planning for re-exploration should begin.

RATIONALE: Intraoperative hypothermia, volume depletion, and blood loss can lead to peripheral vasoconstriction. These patient-specific factors must be assessed and corrected prior to final evaluation of the flap.[6] However, re-exploration should not be delayed as volume is being replaced.

6. A nurse calls you to tell you the flap looks purple and has brisk capillary refill. What do you do?

A congested flap has an outflow (venous) problem, and one must evaluate for venous obstruction. One can try initial maneuvers such as release of sutures, but one should be prepared for emergent return to the operating room.

RATIONALE: Salvage rates are higher for venous obstruction, but venous obstruction will lead to overall flap failure and death more quickly than arterial insufficiency.[2,6,7]

7. Your nonoperative strategies are not successful. What is your operative plan?

Consent the patient for re-exploration, revision of the flap, and possible salvage procedures. First evaluate for external causes of compression, which can be kinking of the vessels, adjacent tissues, hematoma, or proximity of a drain. Once extrinsic causes are excluded, evaluate for intrinsic causes, which include vasospasm. If there is vasospasm, use lidocaine 2% or papaverine 0.25% as an external wash, and then proceed to perform a second anastomosis if possible; if needed, a vein graft can provide a tension-free anastomosis and can bypass injured vessels.

Once extrinsic causes and vasospasm are excluded, evaluate for internal causes, which include early thrombosis (fresh clot) and late thrombosis (established clot). For early thrombosis, it is treated by a heparin flush at a concentration of 100 units/mL with or without a thrombectomy, using a no. 2 or 3 Fogarty catheter. For a late thrombosis (established clot), first heparinize, then perform a thrombectomy, and then use thrombolytics, which include streptokinase and tissue plasminogen activator (TPA). Streptokinase is used at 50,000 to 250,000 units in NS at a concentration of 5,000 units/mL, and TPA is used at 2 to 20 mg at a concentration of 1 mg/mL. The vessel is clamped with an atraumatic clamp proximal to opening, and the vessel is opened. The thrombolytics are infused into an open branch of the artery, left in for 5 to 10 minutes, and allowed to flow out. One then waits for 10 to 15 minutes, and performs the infusion once more (**Fig. 5.2**).

RATIONALE: Authors differ in their dosages of TPA. Rinker et al[8] use 2.5 mg, Casey et al[9] use 2.0 mg, and Bui et al[5] use 5 to 20 mg.

8. When do you decide the free flap will not work?
If one has revised the flap and has been unsuccessful after 6 hours, one aborts the procedure.

9. The flap fails after all of your efforts. What do you do?
There are three options: perform a second free flap, a local flap, or delayed reconstruction. If the patient is medically stable and has exposed vital structures and no local options, a second free flap is performed. If the patient is medically unstable for a second free flap, has exposed vital

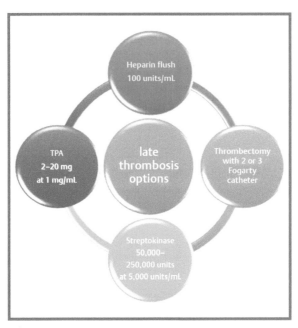

Fig. 5.2 Late thrombosis options.

structures, and does not have recipient vessels, a local flap is performed. If the patient is medically unstable, has no local options, no recipient vessels, and no exposed vital structures, a delayed reconstruction is performed.

References

1. Smit JM, Zeebregts CJ, Acosta R, Werker PMN. Advancements in free flap monitoring in the last decade: a critical review. Plast Reconstr Surg 2010;125(1):177–185
2. Swartz WM, Jones NF, Cherup L, Klein A. Direct monitoring of microvascular anastomoses with the 20-MHz ultrasonic Doppler probe: an experimental and clinical study. Plast Reconstr Surg 1988;81(2):149–161
3. Repez A, Oroszy D, Arnez ZM. Continuous postoperative monitoring of cutaneous free flaps using near infrared spectroscopy. J Plast Reconstr Aesthet Surg 2008;61(1):71–77
4. Budd ME, Evans GRD. Post-operative care. In: Wei F, Mardini S, eds. Flaps, and Reconstructive Surgery. Philadelphia, PA: Saunders Elsevier; 2009:137–143
5. Bui DT, Cordeiro PG, Hu QY, Disa JJ, Pusic A, Mehrara BJ. Free flap reexploration: indications, treatment, and outcomes in 1193 free flaps. Plast Reconstr Surg 2007;119(7):2092–2100
6. Angel MF, Mellow CG, Knight KR, O'Brien BM. Secondary ischemia time in rodents: contrasting complete pedicle interruption with venous obstruction. Plastic and Reconstructive Surgery 1990;85(5):789–793
7. Wilson JL, Morritt AN, Morrison WA. Avoiding complications. In: Wei F, Mardini S, eds. Flaps and Reconstructive Surgery. Philadelphia, PA: Saunders Elsevier; 2009:117–124
8. Rinker BD, Stewart DH, Pu LL, Vasconez HC. Role of recombinant tissue plasminogen activator in free flap salvage. J Reconstr Microsurg 2007;23(2):69–73
9. Casey WJ III, Craft RO, Rebecca AM, Smith AA, Yoon S. Intra-arterial tissue plasminogen activator: an effective adjunct following microsurgical venous thrombosis. Ann Plast Surg 2007;59(5):520–525

6 Fluid Management

Abstract

This chapter will provide information on fluid management of plastic surgery patients, with particular emphasis on liposuction. The reader will be able to plan fluid management in a variety of clinical scenarios, including liposuction, burn, and trauma.

Keywords: postsurgical fluid management, liposuction, trauma, burn

Six Key Points

- Estimate burns by the rule of nines in adults.
- Estimate burns by the Lund and Browder chart in children.
- Fluid resuscitate for greater than 20% body surface area (BSA) burns.
- Resuscitate using 4 mL/kg/% BSA.
- Large-volume liposuction is greater than 4 L.
- For liposuction, fluid ratio is tumescent volume plus intraoperative volume/aspirate.

Questions

General

Case 1

You have just performed an abdominal wall reconstruction on a 56-year-old male with a large ventral hernia.

1. What are the fluid considerations in the perioperative period?
Patients undergoing surgery have both sensible and insensible losses. Sensible losses include those measurable losses such as blood and urine. Insensible losses include respiratory losses and evaporative losses. Some studies have shown that blood volume is not affected by overnight fasting prior to operative procedures.[1] Sensible losses should be replaced on a demand-based regimen. Insensible losses are estimated at 0.5 to 1 mL/kg/h,[2] although some authors do not advocate routine replacement of insensible losses.[3]

Burn

Case 2

A 26-year-old male presents to the emergency department after spilling boiling water on his bilateral hands, abdomen, and thighs.

1. How do you estimate the size of a burn?
Burn size is estimated based on the relative body surface area involved. In pediatric patients, the distribution of body surface area is different than for adults. Wallace's rule of nines assigns percent body surface area in multiples of 9, in which each upper extremity is 9%, each lower extremity is 18%, the front torso is 18%, the back torso is 18%, the head is 9%, and the neck is 1% (see **Fig. 6.1**).

In children, the Lund and Browder chart (**Fig. 6.2**) is often used. It stratifies children based on age (0–1, 1–4, 5–9, 10–14, and 15 years) and reflects the relative larger BSA contributions of the head and torso in the pediatric population.

23

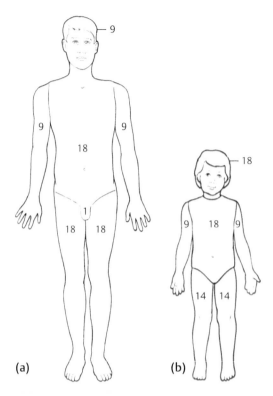

Fig. 6.1 The rule of 9s for estimating a burn size. (Adapted from Lakin GE. Plastic Surgery Review. New York, NY: Thieme; 2015.)

2. How do you fluid resuscitate a burn patient?

Assuming that the patient has been medically stabilized according to Advanced Trauma Life Support (ATLS) guidelines, fluid resuscitation consists of administering crystalloid solution through an IV to patients who have sustained a burn greater than 20% BSA. Lactated Ringer's solution is used for resuscitation and the Parkland formula is a tool for estimating fluid needs in the first 24 hours for an adult.

- The Parkland formula is as follows: 4 mL/kg/% BSA burn.
- Half of the total amount is given in the first 8 hours from the time of injury,

and the second half is given over the next 16 hours.

For pediatric patients, the Galveston formula is used:

- 5,000 mL/m² BSA burn + 2,000 mL/m² total BSA.
- Half of the total amount is given over the first 8 hours from the time of injury and the second half is given over the remaining 16 hours.

3. You start that fluid. How do you know it is adequate?

The adequacy of fluid resuscitation is determined by urine output, which should be at least 0.5 mg/kg/h in adults and 1 mL/kg/h in children.

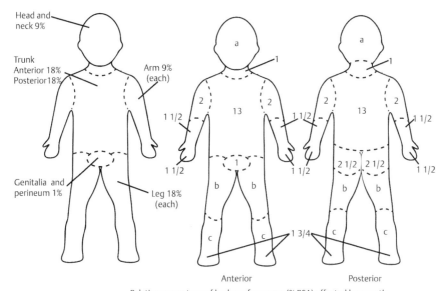

Fig. 6.2 Lund and Browder chart for estimating burn size in children. (Adapted from https://www.remm.nlm.gov/LundBrowder.pdf.)

4. What patient factors will increase fluid need?

Factors associated with increased fluid need are associated trauma, inhalation injury, delay in resuscitation, electrical injuries, and escharotomies.[4]

5. The patient starts to develop edema. What do you do?

One decreases the fluid if urine output is 1.5 mL/kg/h.

6. Why lactated Ringer's solution and not normal saline?

The difference between lactated Ringer's solution and normal saline is the electrolyte composition. One liter of lactated Ringer's solution contains 130 mEq of sodium, 109 mEq of chloride, 28 mEq of lactate, 4 mEq of potassium, and 3 mEq of calcium, while 1L of 0.9% normal saline contains 154 mEq of sodium and 154 mEq of chloride. While they are both considered isotonic, normal saline is near isotonic, and lactated Ringer's solution is isotonic. Large infusions of normal saline can cause a metabolic acidosis. In a swine model of uncontrolled hemorrhagic shock, lactated Ringer's solution was found to be superior to normal saline in resuscitation.[5]

7. Why not colloid?

The albumin in colloid can be associated with pulmonary complications because it can extravasate into the pulmonary interstitium.

Table 6.1 Relationship between liposuction technique, fluid, and blood loss

Liposuction technique	Fluid injected:aspirate	Blood loss
Dry	–	20–45% aspirate
Wet	200–300 mL:–	4–30% aspirate
Superwet	1:1	1% aspirate
Tumescent	3–4:1	1% aspirate

Liposuction

1. How do you define large-volume liposuction LVL?

LVL is that in which the aspirate exceeds 4 L.

2. How do you define wet, superwet, and tumescent techniques of liposuction?

In the wet technique, 200 to 300 mL is injected in each area. In the superwet technique, the fluid is injected in a 1:1 ratio with the aspirate. In the tumescent technique, fluid is injected with a 3:1 to 4:1 ratio with the aspirate (**Table 6.1**).

3. What are your clinical concerns in fluid management in LVL?

In LVL, a significant amount of the tumescent solution (60–80%) can remain in the tissue and be absorbed. Large fluid shifts can occur, and the most concerning sequela of LVL is fluid overload, which can lead to pulmonary edema or congestive heart failure.

4. What is the "fluid ratio" method for managing intraoperative volume?

The fluid ratio refers to tumescent fluid volume plus intraoperative volume divided by the volume of aspirate.[6,7] The general aim is to keep the fluid ratio 1:1 and a urine output of 1 to 1.5 mL/kg/h.

5. What is the recipe for tumescent fluid?

One liter of lactated Ringer's solution with 1 ampule of epinephrine (1:1,000), and 20 mL of 2% lidocaine. This gives a concentration of epinephrine of 1:1,000,000 and a 0.04% lidocaine solution.

6. What is the maximum dose of lidocaine?

In the tumescent liposuction technique, doses of up to 50 mg/kg can be used, which is considered off-label usage.

Websites

http://www.utmb.edu/pedi_ed/CORE/Fluids&Electyrolytes/page_04.htm

http://www.ncbi.nlm.nih.gov/pmc/articles/PMC3141144

http://drtrott.com/news/safety-considerations-and-fluid-resuscitation-in-liposuction-an-analysis-of-53-consecutive-patients/

http://scholar.google.com/scholar_url?url=http://anesthesiology.pubs.asahq.org/data/Journals/JASA/931047/0000542-200810000-00021.pdf&hl=en&sa=X&scisig=AAGBfm0m3AODb8ckRjWIbG-WiCHf_LAr3Aw&nossl=1&oi=scholarr

References

1. Jacob M, Chappell D, Conzen P, Finsterer U, Rehm M. Blood volume is normal after preoperative overnight fasting. Acta Anaesthesio Scand 2008;52(4):522–529

2. Lamke LO, Nilsson GE, Reithner HL. Water loss by evaporation from the abdominal cavity during surgery. Acta Chir Scand 1977;143(5):279–284, as cited in Chappell

3. Chappell D, Jacob M, Hofmann-Kiefer K, Conzen P, Rehm M. A rational approach

to perioperative fluid management. Anesthesiology 2008;109(4):723–740

4. Smith CR, Cobb JP. Thermal injuries. In: Doherty GM, Meko JB, Olson JA, Peplinski GR, Worrall NK, eds. The Washington Manual of Surgery. 2nd ed. Philadelphia, PA: Lippincott Williams & Wilkins; 1999

5. Todd SR, Malinoski D, Muller PJ, Schreiber MA. Lactated Ringer's is superior to normal saline in the resuscitation of uncontrolled hemorrhagic shock. J Trauma 2007;62(3):636–639

6. Trott SA, Beran SJ, Rohrich RJ, Kenkel JM, Adams WP Jr, Klein KW. Safety considerations and fluid resuscitation in liposuction: an analysis of 53 consecutive patients. Plast Reconstr Surg 1998;102(6):2220–2229

7. Thomas M, Bhorkar N, D'Silva J, Menon H, Bandekar N. Anesthesia considerations in large-volume lipoplasty. Aesthet Surg J 2007;27(6):607–611

7 Ethical Considerations

Abstract

This chapter will review common ethical principles and their applications in plastic surgery. The reader will be able to assess the ethical considerations in ethical dilemmas likely to appear on the plastic surgery oral board examination and in practice, and resolve those using ethical principles.

Keywords: biomedical ethics, ethics, principlism

Six Key Points

- Modern bioethics relies on principlism.
- Any given issue can have different resolution depending on application of principles.
- Decision-making capacity is dynamic and can be assessed by a clinician.
- Using reviews to influence surgical decision-making is unethical.
- Financial contracts should be arranged prior to surgery.
- Different societies have different guidelines.

Overview

Ethical considerations in plastic surgery tend to manifest in three ways: billing/coding, decisions to operate, and informed consent.

Ethics in billing and coding requires an attention to detail and continual education in coding practices. The American Society of Plastic Surgeons provides resources for coding. General principles include avoiding unbundling and avoiding upcoding. It is important to remember that while systematic upcoding is potentially fraudulent, so too is downcoding.

The principles of bioethics underpin decisions to operate and informed consent. There are seven basic rights of patients—three negative rights and four positive rights. Negative rights include the following: not to be killed intentionally or negligently by the surgeon, not to be harmed by intent or negligence of the surgeon, and not to be deceived by the surgeon. Positive rights include the following: to be adequately informed of the risks and benefits of surgery; to be treated by a knowledgeable, competent practitioner; to have his health more highly valued than the surgeon's economic interest; and to decide whether to accept treatment under the conditions described.[1]

The principlism approach to biomedical ethics has four principles as its underpinning respect for autonomy, nonmaleficence, beneficence, and justice (**Fig. 7.1**). A casuistic approach is a heuristic approach of ethical analysis, originally performed by Jesuits—this case-based approach is still used today. In this approach, underlying principles include the indications for medical intervention, patient preference, quality-of-life concerns, and contextual features.

Autonomy requires that the surgeon identifies the patient's values and beliefs, respects their role in the patient's life, and elicits the patient's preferences from among

28

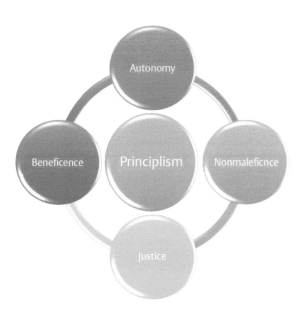

Fig. 7.1 The principlism approach to bioethics. Foundations are autonomy, beneficence, nonmalefi- cence, and justice. Note that these principles can lead to different conclusions about a given bioethical issue de- pending on which takes the foreground.

the medical and surgical alternatives sup- ported in beneficence-based clinical judg- ment. Beneficence requires that the surgeon act in ways that are reliably expected to result in a greater balance of clinical goods over harms for the patient. A classic exam- ple of the intersection of autonomy and beneficence is blood transfusions in the Jehovah's Witness population.

Nonmaleficence is manifested in a refusal to perform surgery. While justice does not usually come into play in the day- to-day decision-making of plastic sur- geons, the allocation of limited financial, material, and human resources is a consid- eration in the broader delivery of health care. Current concepts of justice include egalitarian, in which patients are treated as equally as possible in the process of care, redistributive, in which universal access is considered a priority, and libertarian, in which justice is achieved by providing patients with adequate information, which creates a level playing field.

Informed consent requires that there is a disclosure to the patient of adequate, clear information about the patient's diagnosis, the patient understands that information, and the patient has a process of deci- sion-making, based not only on what the surgeon has told him, but also on informa- tion from other sources.

According to the Professional Practice Standards, the patient is told what an experienced physician would tell the patient. According to the reasonable per- son standard, the patient is told all of the information a reasonable person would need to make a decision.

The seven steps of informed consent are tell the patient about the process of informed consent, elicit the patient's understanding of the problem, elaborate on options (using a reasonable person standard), assist the patient in developing cognitive understanding, assist the patient in evaluating the alternatives available, offer a recommendation, and the patient finally articulates a decision for or against surgery.

Decision-making capacity describes an ability to understand and appreciate the nature and consequences of health decisions and to formulate and communicate decisions concerning health care. Decision-making capacity has four components: the capacity to communicate choices, the capacity to understand relevant information, the capacity to appreciate the situation and its consequences, and the capacity to manipulate information rationally. It is important to note that decision-making capacity is a clinical judgment, rather than a legal one, and is a dynamic, rather than a static state. A clinician can—and should—determine whether a patient has decision-making capacity for any given decision. For example, a patient who arrives to the ER with a high blood alcohol level, with visible signs of inebriation, may not have decision-making capacity at that time, but may have decision-making capacity when he is sober (see text box below).

Ten myths of decision-making capacity

- Decision-making capacity (DMC) and legal competency are the same.
- Lack of DMC is a permanent condition.
- Lack of DMC can be presumed when patients go against medical advice.
- Patients with misinformation lack DMC.
- There is no need to assess DMC unless patients go against medical advice.
- Patients with certain psychiatric disorders lack DMC.
- Patients who are involuntarily committed lack DMC.
- DMC is all or nothing.
- Cognitive impairment equals lack of DMC.
- Only mental health experts can assess DMC.

Clinical equipoise is used in research, and is used to describe the concept that if the clinician knows, or has good reason to believe, that a new therapy (A) is better than another therapy (B), he cannot participate in a comparative trial of therapy A versus therapy B. Ethically, the physician is obligated to give therapy A to each new patient with a need for one of these therapies. The requirement for clinical equipoise is satisfied if there is uncertainty in the medical community.

It is important to understand, when discussing ethical issues in plastic surgery, that the lens through which one views the particular ethical questions (beneficence or autonomy, e.g.), can result in different but equally valid conclusions. Consider Case 1, in which two diffrent answers are presented.

Questions

Case 1

1. You offer a woman a facelift and laser treatment for an aging face. She would like products for skin care. Do you sell them to her out of your office?

Answer 1: No. The American College of Physicians has a position against physicians selling products out of their offices, unless certain conditions are met, such as medical necessity and urgency (e.g., splinting equipment), sufficient evidence to justify their use medically, full disclosure of the financial benefit to the physician, and encouragement by the physician to the patient to find cheaper alternatives. In the case of skin care products, they are likely to be neither emergent nor unavailable elsewhere, and the physician who sells them is using his position to financially benefit from the trust of his patient.

Answer 2: Yes. Selling products out of the office affords patients some convenience. The criteria of informed consent and patient autonomy are met by transparency in pricing, and discussion of alternatives.

Case 2

1. You perform a facelift on a patient, and she is unsatisfied. She would like her money back. What do you tell her?

All office policies on pricing and refunds are laid out in the preoperative financial forms, which patients sign prior to the procedure. If the office policy is to not provide refunds, she does not get a refund. It is reasonable to work with her and discuss the specifics of her dissatisfaction with the results, and assess whether further intervention would help, and whether her expectations from the original procedure were realistic. It is advisable to also review her preoperative photographs with her postoperative photographs.

2. She states she is going to go online and write a bad review of you if you don't give her money back. How do you respond?

It is always an option for patients to go online and write reviews, bad or good. Reviews—good or bad—are not appropriately used as bargaining chips for financial transactions in a surgery practice.

References

1. Beauchamp TL, Childress JF. Principles of Biomedical Ethics. 6th ed. Oxford: Oxford University Press; 2008

8 Skin Cancer

Abstract

This chapter will review the workup and management of skin cancer, including basal cell carcinoma, squamous cell carcinoma, and melanoma. The reader will develop preoperative workup plans for these cancers, describe cancer staging, and generate surgical plans for their resection, including oncologic margin control.

Keywords: skin cancer, nonmelanoma skin cancer, squamous cell carcinoma, basal cell carcinoma, keratoacanthoma

Six Key Points

- Skin lesions need a tissue diagnosis.
- Treatment of basal cell carcinoma is dependent on whether the lesion is high risk or low risk.
- Skin malignancies need oncologic margins.
- Complete circumferential peripheral and deep margin assessment can be used when Mohs is not available.
- Melanoma must be staged.
- Treatment of melanoma depends on stage.

Questions

Case 1

A patient has a lesion of his left cheek (**Fig. 8.1**).

1. What is your differential diagnosis?

Skin lesions are described using the ABCDE scheme. Asymmetry, borders, color, diameter, and elevation. This provides a unified description pattern. While the differential diagnosis of all skin lesions is quite large, lesions are either benign or malignant. The most common benign lesions include seborrheic keratosis, nevus sebaceous, epidermal nevus, and actinic keratosis.

2. How do you distinguish between the different benign skin lesions clinically?

- **Seborrheic keratoses:** Seborrheic keratoses have a waxy, "stuck-on" appearance and have well-demarcated borders. Over time, they can develop darker brown pigment. They typically occur on the face, neck, and trunk.
- **Actinic keratosis:** Actinic keratosis (also known as solar keratosis) has a sandpaper feel and is usually several millimeters, but can be larger (**Fig. 8.2**).
- **Nevus sebaceous:** Nevus sebaceous is a hairless verrucous plaque, and occurs most commonly on the scalp and face. While malignant transformation is rare, it can occur and surgical excision of these lesions is recommended in suspicious cases (**Fig. 8.3**).
- **Epidermal Nevus:** An epidermal nevus typically appears in the first year of life as a well-circumscribed plaque, most commonly on the trunk or extremities.
- **Melanocytic Nevi:** Melanocytic nevi are pigmented and can be congenital, acquired, or atypical. They can occur anywhere on the body.

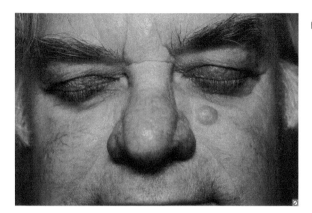

Fig. 8.1 Lesion of left cheek.

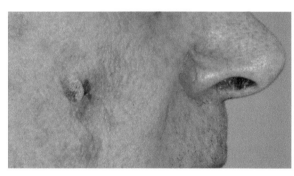

Fig. 8.2 Actinic keratosis. While they are usually small, note that they can be larger.

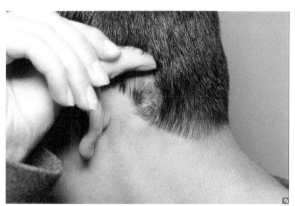

Fig. 8.3 Nevus sebaceous. The scalp location is quite common.

3. How should a keratoacanthoma be treated?

A keratoacanthoma has a distinctive course and appearance. It is a fast-growing lesion that has an ulcerated center (**Fig. 8.4**).

A traditional shave or punch biopsy is not recommended for a keratoacanthoma because of the difficulty in distinguishing it from squamous cell carcinoma.

4. What are the malignant skin lesions?

The malignant skin lesions are subdivided into melanoma and nonmelanoma skin cancer and nonmelanoma skin

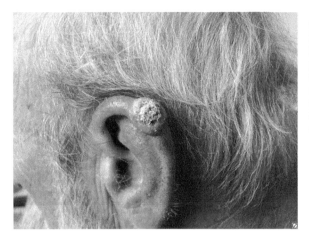

Fig. 8.4 Example of a lesion consistent with keratoacanthoma. The patient reported a history of fast growth, over the course of 2 months. Final pathology on excisional biopsy demonstrated invasive squamous cell carcinoma.

cancer include basal cell carcinomas and squamous cell carcinomas.

5. How do you biopsy it?

While basal cell carcinomas (BCCs) and squamous cell carcinomas can have accurate diagnoses by shave biopsy, melanoma requires a punch biopsy to determine depth. An incisional biopsy allows diagnoses of BCC and squamous cell carcinoma, with the exception of a keratoacanthoma as above.

6. The diagnosis is a BCC. What do you do?

Treatment for BCC is determined by the specific characteristics of a given BCC, including size, location, and histological features. Treatment options include electrodessication and curettage, topical and (less commonly) intralesional agents, photodynamic therapy, radiation therapy, Mohs surgery, and surgical excision (**Fig. 8.5**).

7. Describe each of these therapies.

Electrodessication and curettage is used for low-risk tumors because histology is not performed and margins cannot be assessed. There are no randomized controlled trials of this technique, and recurrence rates vary from 6 to 19%[1] (**Fig. 8.6**).

Topical agents include imiquimod 5% cream, approved for treatment of low-risk superficial and nodular BCC. Topical 5-fluorouracil (5-FU; 5%) does not have randomized controlled trials proving its efficacy but is often used in low-risk, superficial BCCs.

Intralesional agents including interferons, 5-FU, and bleomycin can be used. Of these, only interferons have randomized controlled trials.[2] Because of lower cure rates and unknown efficacy, these therapies are used for high-risk lesions in nonsurgical candidates.

Photodynamic therapy involves placement of a photosensitizing porphyrin on the lesion, followed by the application of visible light in the 40- to 450- or 630- to 635-nm range. It is used on superficial lesions.

Radiation therapy is reserved for patients who cannot tolerate surgical intervention.

Mohs surgery is used for high-risk lesions or lesions in cosmetically or functionally sensitive areas. It is generally not recommended for low-risk lesions or those on the trunk or extremities, because the time and expense of Mohs is not justified.

Surgical excision requires oncologic margins. Because BCCs are contiguous lesions, oncological margins are simply

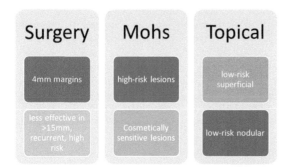

Fig. 8.5 Treatment options for basal cell carcinoma

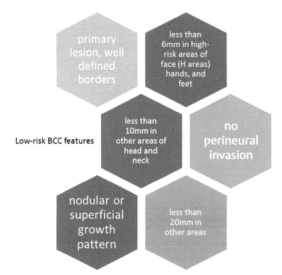

Fig. 8.6 Low-risk basal cell carcinoma features.

cancer-free margins. Because of the way pathology is read, however, oncological margins require several millimeters. The majority of studies have looked at 2- to 5-mm margins, and recurrence rate for 5-mm margins is 0.4% and that for 4-mm margins is 1.6%. Features that will decrease cure rates include size of primary BCC greater than 15 mm, lesions in high-risk areas, and recurrent tumors (**Fig. 8.7**).

margins. One has the option of performing en face margin assessment at the time of surgery and reconstruction, or waiting for permanent sections and performing reconstruction when permanent pathology is available. In either case, it is important to counsel the patient of the fact that more surgery may be needed if final margins are positive. The ultimate oncologic plan is based on the type and location of the BCC (**Fig. 8.8**).

8. The lesion is in a high-risk area of the face, but there is no Mohs surgeon available. What do you do?

If no Mohs' surgeon is available, one performs surgical resection with 4-mm

9. The diagnosis is a squamous cell carcinoma. What do you do?

A surgical excision can be performed with permanent sections and delayed repair, or excision with 3- to 4-mm margins.

The first-line treatment is surgical excision with oncologic margin control. While no randomized controlled trials have been performed, current recommendations are for a minimal margin of at least 5 mm.[3]

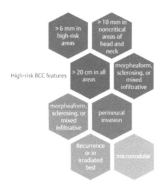

Fig. 8.7 High-risk basal cell carcinoma features.

If the lesion has a thickness of greater than 6 mm, or if the tumor has high-risk features (**Fig. 8.8**), a margin of 10 mm is recommended.[3]

The involvement of lymph nodes is a predictor of recurrence as well as mortality. A lymph node ultrasound is recommended for tumors with high-risk characteristics. If there is a suspicious lymph node, a fine needle aspiration or biopsy is recommended.

10. There is evidence that there is at least one involved lymph node. What do you do?
There is no evidence that a sentinel lymph node biopsy has meaningful prognostic or therapeutic value, and there is no indication for a sentinel lymph node biopsy. If there is evidence of involvement of the lymph nodes, I would perform a full regional lymph node dissection.

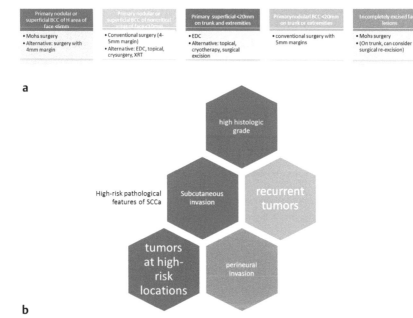

Fig. 8.8 (**a**) Treatment of basal cell carcinoma by type. (**b**) High-risk pathological features of squamous cell carcinoma.

11. The patient is a poor surgical candidate. What do you do?

Because radiation therapy has some utility in the treatment of cutaneous squamous cell carcinoma, referral to radiationoncology is appropriate. Other indications for radiation therapy are tumors that are inoperable or are in low-risk areas.

12. What are the indications for further workup?

If there are signs of involvement with underlying or adjacent structures, further imaging is recommended.

13. The lesion is near the eye. What other imaging would you get, and why or why not?

I would get an MRI (preferentially) or a CT scan. An MRI will help delineate the involvement of other structures, and will help predict whether an orbital exenteration will be indicated.

Case 2

A patient presents with a biopsy-proven melanoma of the forearm.

1. What do you do?

The first step in management is to accurately stage the melanoma. Melanoma is staged with the TNM (tumor size, node involvement, and metastasis status) system. The tumor (T) is assessed by Breslow's thickness (**Table 8.1**).

2. What are the margins you take?

Margins are determined by depth of thickness of the melanoma (**Fig. 8.9a,b**).

3. The patient has metastatic disease. What do you do?

If there are only a few sites of metastases, one can consider surgical excision for local control. Otherwise, patients are candidates for systemic therapy with checkpoint-inhibitor immunotherapy and therapy

Table 8.1 Melanoma staging

Stage	Criteria
0	Confined to epidermis, melanoma in situ
1A	< 1 mm thick, no ulceration
1B	< 1 mm thick with ulceration; 1–2 mm thick without ulceration
2A	1–2 mm thick with ulceration; 2–4 mm thick without ulceration
2B	2–4 mm thick with ulceration; > 4 mm thick without ulceration
2C	> 4 mm thick with ulceration
3A	Any thickness, without ulceration; 3 or fewer affected lymph nodes with microscopic disease
3B	Ulcerated, 1–3 lymph nodes with microscopic disease OR without ulceration, 1–3 lymph nodes with macroscopic disease OR without ulceration, skin but not lymph node involvement
3C	Skip lesions and lymph node involvement OR ulceration and 1–3 lymph nodes with macroscopic disease OR with or without ulceration and > 4 lymph nodes involved OR with or without ulceration and joined involved lymph nodes
4	Metastatic disease

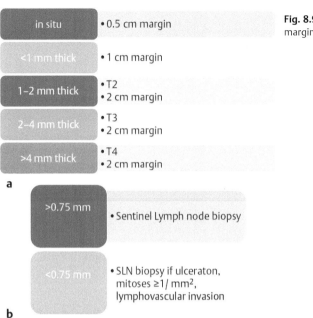

Fig. 8.9 Recommended margins for melanoma.

against the mitogen activated protein kinase pathway.

References

1. Thissen MR, Neumann MH, Schouten LJ. A systematic review of treatment modalities for primary basal cell carcinomas. Arch Dermatol 1999;135(10):1177–1183

2. Kirby JS, Miller CJ. Intralesional chemotherapy for nonmelanoma skin cancer. J Am Acad Dermatol 2010;63: 689–702

3. Stratigos A, Garbe C, Lebbe C, et al; European Dermatology Forum (EDF); European Association of Dermato-Oncology (EADO); European Organization for Research and Treatment of Cancer (EORTC). Diagnosis and treatment of invasive squamous cell carcinoma of the skin: European consensus-based interdisciplinary guideline. Eur J Cancer 2015;51(14):1989–2007

9 Reconstruction of the Facial Defect

Abstract

This chapter will review reconstructive options for reconstruction of the eyelids, ears, nose, cheek, and mouth. It will be linked to drawing/photographs in an appendix for reader practice of flap design and marking. The reader will evaluate the defect and prioritize flaps for the reconstruction of eyelid, ear, nose, cheek, and lip defects.

Keywords: facial defect, eyelids reconstruction, ear reconstruction, nose reconstruction, cheek reconstruction, lip reconstruction

Six Key Points

- Characterize all facial defects by size and involved lamellae.
- Reconstruction will be based on size and involved lamellae by algorithm.
- Always await final pathology prior to reconstruction.
- If final pathology is not known, many defects can be temporized with skin grafts.
- The majority of defects can be managed with local or regional flaps.
- Know at least two options for any given defect.

Questions

Eyelid Reconstruction

Case 1

A 47-year-old woman comes for discussion of eyelid reconstruction after excision of a resection of a basal cell carcinoma.

1. What are your reconstructive goals?
Reconstructive goals in the eyelid are threefold: to restore the height and length components of the eyelid, to restore the function of globe protection, and to avoid complications, such as tethering, that reverse or prevent accomplishment of structural and mechanical restoration.

2. How do you analyze the defect?
Analysis is systematic, and considers the etiology, which includes assessment of zone of injury (ZOI), the anatomic defect, and the available tissues for reconstruction. The etiology includes senescent changes, traumatic defects both controlled (such as surgical defects for tumor extirpation) and traumatic. In addition, there are both acute and chronic ZOI considerations. An acute ZOI consideration is a traction injury, which may damage the canaliculi. A chronic ZOI consideration is previous radiation or periorbital surgery, or senescent changes, which may affect reconstructive options (**Fig. 9.1**).

The anatomic defect must be assessed in both the medial–lateral extent and the superficial to deep extent, which includes the bilamellae, the lacrimal drainage system, and the ligamentous support of the eyelid ("tarsoligamentous sling").[1] The anterior lamella of the upper and lower lids contains the skin and orbicularis muscle. The middle lamella contains the orbital septum, fat, and eyelid retractors. The posterior lamella contains the tarsal plate and the nonkeratinized conjunctiva.

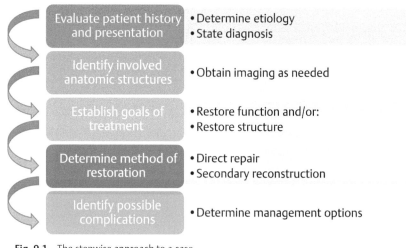

Evaluate patient history and presentation
• Determine etiology
• State diagnosis

Identify involved anatomic structures
• Obtain imaging as needed

Establish goals of treatment
• Restore function and/or:
• Restore structure

Determine method of restoration
• Direct repair
• Secondary reconstruction

Identify possible complications
• Determine management options

Fig. 9.1   The stepwise approach to a case.

3. How might senescent changes or previous surgery affect reconstructive options?

In general, the percentage of the eyelid that is affected is a major determinant of the type of reconstruction performed. Scarred or irradiated tissue may have decreased laxity, which may mean that only smaller defects can be reconstructed with certain methods. Similarly, increased laxity may mean that larger defects can be reconstructed.

4. There is a partial-thickness defect of the lid. How do you repair it?

The approach to reconstruction needs to include the anterior lamella and the posterior lamella. The anterior lamella can be reconstructed with a skin graft, assuming there is an adequate bed. Full-thickness skin graft donor sites can be excess eyelid skin, preauricular or posterior auricular skin, or supraclavicular skin.

5. The defect is a full-thickness defect that is 20% of the lower lid. What do you do?

For full-thickness defects of the lower or upper lid that are less than 25% of the lid, the lid can be directly closed. The edges

can be cut into a pentagonal configuration (**Fig. 9.2**) and the lid edge is closed with 6–0 sutures that come out through the gray line, the tarsal plate is repaired with 6–0 chromic, and the skin is closed with 5–0 fast gut suture.

6. As you attempt to close the lid, it doesn't quite reach without tension. What do you do?

A lateral canthotomy can be performed if the tissues appear to have tension, and are often required with defects 20 to 30% of the lid length. The canthotomy site is closed with suture to create a sharp canthal angle, and if a canthopexy can be performed, it is.

7. The lateral eyelid appears loose. What do you do?

A canthopexy can be performed.

8. The defect is 50% of the upper lid. What do you do?

A Tenzel semicircular flap.

9. Draw it.

The drawing is shown in **Fig. 9.3**.

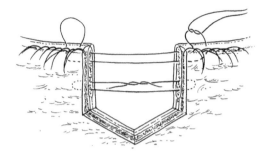

Fig. 9.2 Pentagonal configuration of lower lid cuts for a closure. (From Chen WP. Oculoplastic Surgery: The Essentials. New York, NY: Thieme Medical Publishers; 2001.)

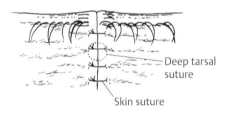

Deep tarsal suture

Skin suture

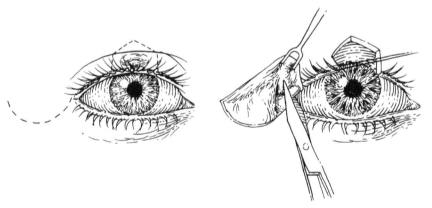

Fig. 9.3 Tenzel's semicircular flap. (From Chen WP. Oculoplastic Surgery: The Essentials. New York, NY: Thieme Medical Publishers; 2001.)

10. The patient has a prior canthotomy. Can you still perform the Tenzel flap?

No. The Tenzel skin–muscle flap requires an intact lateral canthal tendon.

11. The defect is 75% of the upper lid. What do you do?

A lid-sharing flap such as a Cutler–Beard flap is appropriate.

12. Describe the flap and draw it.

The Cutler–Beard flap can be used for rectangular defects and takes skin, orbicularis muscle, and conjunctive from the lower lid. A cartilage graft to replace the tarsal defect can be sandwiched between the layers of the graft and sutured into place (**Fig. 9.4**).

13. The defect is 75% of the lower lid. What do you do?

A Hughes tarsoconjunctival flap can reconstruct defects greater than two-thirds of the lower lid.

14. Describe the flap and draw it.

The Hughes tarsoconjunctival flap is designed on the conjunctival surface of the upper lid. A rectangle is created on the conjunctival surface of the upper lid, at least 3 mm cranial to the lid margin. The dissection can include Muller's muscle or not, and the dissection proceeds from caudal to cranial including the tarsal plate. Once the flap is freed, it is advanced and sutured into the conjunctiva and lower lid retractors. This reconstruction addresses the posterior lamellae; the anterior lamella needs to be covered with either a skin graft or an advancement flap (**Fig. 9.5**).

15. When do you divide the flap?

The flap is divided between 4 and 6 weeks. It is divided slightly more cranial than the margin to allow for retraction.

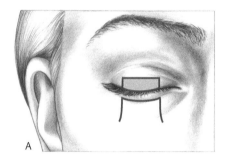

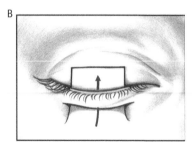

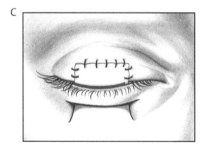

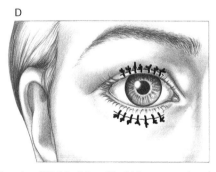

Fig. 9.4   Cutler–Beard flap. (From Sherris DA, Larrabee WF. Principles of Facial Reconstruction: A Subunite Approach to Cutaneous Repair. New York, NY: Thieme Medical Publishers; 2009.)

16. After you divide the flap, you notice elevation of the upper lid. What do you do?
Under anesthesia, you can evert the upper eyelid and divide bands of scar.

17. The lower lid is too high. What do you do?
Direct excision of the lower lid can reduce the height.

The posterior lamella can be reconstructed with a tarsoconjunctival graft.

18. Describe how you take the tarsoconjunctival graft.
The tarsoconjunctival graft is taken from the upper lid. At least 4 mm of the caudal border of the tarsus is left in situ to maintain integrity of the upper lid tarsus, and 2 mm of conjunctiva is harvested on the superior border—this is used to reconstruct the lid margin. The donor site heals by secondary intention.

19. That fails. What do you do?
A hard palate mucoperiosteal graft is a secondary option for posterior lamella reconstruction.

20. Why wasn't it your first choice?
The donor site morbidity is more significant with a hard palate graft than with a

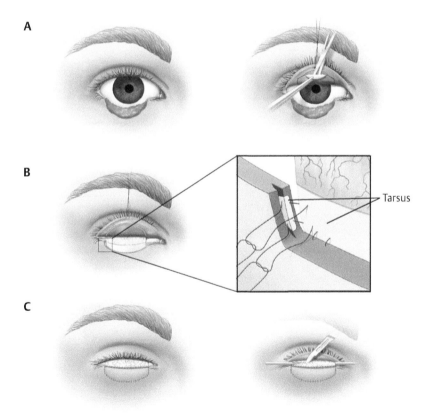

Fig. 9.5 Hughes tarsoconjunctival flap. (From Janis JE. Essentials of Plastic Surgery. 2nd ed. New York, NY: Thieme Medical Publishers; 2014.)

tarsoconjunctival graft, and there is a potential for corneal irritation from the epithelium of a hard palate graft.

21. You can't harvest hard palate mucoperiosteum. What other graft options do you have?

Nasal chondromucosal and auricular cartilage.

22. What other options are there for reconstruction?

A tarsomarginal graft can be used which is a 7- to 8-mm, wedge-shaped composite graft of the tarsus, conjunctiva, and lid margin. Once this is placed, the anterior lamella is covered with a myocutaneous flap.

23. She comes back 1 year later and complains that she has no eyelashes. What do you tell her?

Part of the initial discussion is that eyelashes may not survive on a tarsomarginal graft.

Upper Eyelid Reconstruction

Case 2

After Mohs resection, a patient has a defect that is 20% of the upper lid.

1. What do you do?

A 20% defect of the upper lid can be repaired primarily. If there is significant laxity, as in the elderly, larger defects can be repaired with direct closure, and cantholysis can increase the percentage defect to 50%.

2. The defect of the upper lid is 50 to 60%. What do you do?

The Tenzel semicircular flap is a great option for defects ranging from 40 to 60% of both upper and lower lids (Table 9.1).

Ear Reconstruction

1. Describe your approach to the ear defect.

The ear is first assessed regarding the structures of the ear that are involved. This principle does not apply to If there is pre-existing pathology, such as effacement of the antihelical fold, prominence of the concha—both of which may lead to a prominent ear—this is assessed. Asymmetry of the ear is also assessed. Finally, the amount of defect is estimated as a percentage of the ear.

The helical rim, sulcus, and antihelical fold are evaluated as subunits of the ear.

2. A patient presents after resection of a basal cell carcinoma of the helical rim. The defect measures 1.5 cm. What do you do?

A helical rim defect that measures 2 cm or less can be closed with an Antia–Buch flap.

Table 9.1   Reconstruction of eyelid defects by location and size

	Less than one-third	One-third to two-thirds	Greater than two-thirds
Upper lid defect	Direct closure	Direct closure with lateral cantholysis; local or other regional options	Cutler–Beard flap
Lower lid defect	Direct closure	Direct closure with lateral cantholysis; semicircular flap (Tenzel); semicircular flap with periosteal flap	Tarsoconjunctival flap (Hughes)

3. Describe it and draw it.

An incision is made along the anterior border of the helical rim, extending to the root of the helix in the concha. The two edges of the helical defect are advanced and the incision is closed (**Fig. 9.6**).

4. The A.ntia–Buch flap separated and you have exposed perichondrium. What do you do?

The Antia–Buch flap can be readvanced, or a full-thickness skin graft can be placed over the defect.

5. The defect included the antihelical fold. Can you still perform an Antia–Buch flap?

No. Depending on the defect, it can be converted to a wedge excision and closed primarily.

6. How do you counsel the patient about these procedures?

It is important that the patient understand that in both of the procedures the ear is made smaller.

7. The defect is 20% of the helical length. What do you do?

An option is to use a conchal cartilage graft, provided that at least one of the helical rim, antihelical fold, or sulcus is intact.

8. The defect is greater than 25% of the helical length. What do you do?

A rib cartilage graft is used.

9. There is a near-total def.ect of the ear. What do you dwo?

A near-total defect of the ear requires reconstruction with a *structural framework* and a *skin envelope.* The structural framework is obtained from rib cartilage, in which the contralateral rib cartilage is harvested and shaped into a base and a helical rim. The framework is placed into a pocket and covered with a temporoparietal flap, and a skin graft (**Table 9.2**).

Nose Reconstruction

1. How do you analyze a defect of the nose?

The defect of the nose is assessed as a combination of the percentage of each

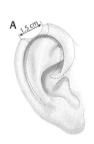 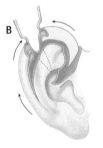 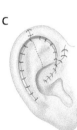

Fig. 9.6 Antia–Buch flap. (From Woo AS. Plastic Surgery Case Review: Oral Board Study Guide. New York, NY: Thieme Medical Publishers; 2014.)

Table 9.2 Reconstruction of ear defects by size

Defect size	Reconstruction	Alternative
< 2 cm	Antia–Buch flap	Wedge excision
< 25% helical length	Conchal cartilage graft	
> 25% helical length	Rib cartilage	
Total or near-total defect	Brent's four-stage reconstruction	Brent two-stage reconstruction
Intact perichondrium	Full-thickness skin graft	

aesthetic subunit that is affected, and the anatomic structures that are involved, specifically, the cover (skin), support (cartilage or bone), and lining (mucosa).

2. What does the percentage matter for each subunit?

If more than 50% of a convex subunit is involved, the rest of the subunit is excised and the entirety of the subunit is reconstructed. This principle does not apply to concave subunits. The determination of reconstructive technique takes into consideration subunit and size of the defect (**Table 9.3**).

3. How do you stage a nose reconstruction in a complex facial reconstruction that also requires reconstruction of other areas of the face?

The nose should be reconstructed last, on a stable base.

4. What materials are used for each subunit?

For lining, septal mucosal turnover flaps, mucoperichondrial flaps, skin grafts, and free flaps can be used. For support, septal, rib, or auricular cartilage can be used, and if bone is needed harvest sites include rib, calvarial bone, and iliac bone. The skin cover can be created with local flaps, skin grafts, and regional or free flaps (**Table 9.4**).

5. You perform a composite graft, and the graft appears dusky 2 weeks post-op. What do you do?

I would manage it conservatively.

6. He or she wants you to intervene. What do you tell him or her?

Even a dusky graft may survive, and part of the graft may survive. I would continue to manage it conservatively.

Table 9.3 Reconstruction of nose defects by location and size

Defect location	Size	Management	Technique	Notes
Nasal tip	< 0.5 cm	Direct closure	6–0 nylon	
Medial canthus, nasal sidewall	Any	Full-thickness skin graft	Posterior auricular, supraclavicular, consider forehead	
Alae	< 1 cm	Composite graft	Conchal cartilage, helical root	
Tip, ala, sidewall	1.5 cm	Bilobed flap		
Alae, nasal sidewall	Any size	Nasolabial	V-Y advancement or interpolation flap	Can base superiorly or inferiorly (can also augment with structural support)
Nasal tip (midline)	2.5 cm	Dorsal nasal flap		Some contour deformity expected
Large defect, multiple units	Any size	Forehead flap		

Table 9.4 Uses of cartilage grafts in nasal reconstruction

Type of cartilage	Use
Septal	Columellar strut, dorsal buttress, nasal sidewall
Auricular cartilage	Alar support, tip definition
Costal	Columellar strut, dorsal buttress

7. The patient has a large defect and you perform a forehead flap. Describe how you do it.

In the first stage, the flap is created and inset (**Fig. 9.7**). In the second stage, 3 weeks later, the flap is debulked and thinned, and the structural support is placed. In the third stage, the flap is divided and inset.

A template of the defect is made using paper or suture wrapper. The supratrochlear vessels are Dopplered with a handheld pencil Doppler and the base of the pedicle is centered over the vessel with a width of approximately 1.5 cm. The flap is designed using the template and the distance is verified using a piece of string. The flap is elevated initially thin, and periosteum is left at the base of the flap.

The flap is inset. The donor site is closed directly and the exposed pedicle is managed with Vaseline gauze.

8. The patient returns 3 months later and states he or she is unhappy with the scar. What options can you offer him or her?

He or she can have dermabrasion for the scarring. I would offer it after 1 year.

Cheek Reconstruction

1. How do you analyze the defect?

The defect is analyzed based on the aesthetic zone of the cheek (suborbital, preauricular, and buccomandibular; **Fig. 9.8**) and the layers and structures involved, including skin, subcutaneous tissue, parotid gland, and facial nerve, and patient-specific

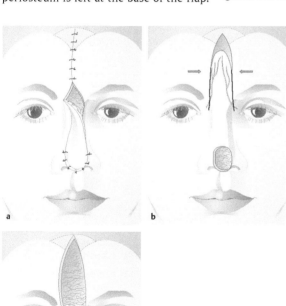

Fig. 9.7 forehead flap. From Weerda H. Reconstructive Facial Plastic Surgery: A Problem-Solving Manual. Stuttgart, Germany: Thieme Medical Publishers; 2015.

features, such as surrounding laxity and other scars.

2. What are your reconstructive goals?

Reconstructive goals are control of the wound, and maintenance of or restoration of oral competence.

3. The defect is 4 cm after a cancer resection. What do you do?

The first concern is oncological clearance. Assuming that the pathology is final and the margins are clear, a defect of up to 4 cm can be closed primarily with wide undermining.

4. The defect is 6 cm, and the final pathology is not back. What do you do?

I would place a temporary skin graft on the area, and perform definitive reconstruction once the final pathology is back and the margins are clear. This has two advantages: first, it provides stable coverage of the wound, and in some cases, if patients decide they do not want further intervention, the reconstructive process is complete. Second, it does not burn a reconstructive bridge, but helps prevent wound contraction that may lead to distortion of features.

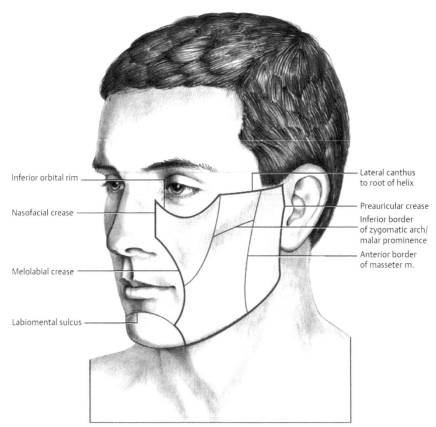

Inferior orbital rim

Nasofacial crease

Melolabial crease

Labiomental sulcus

Lateral canthus to root of helix

Preauricular crease

Inferior border of zygomatic arch/ malar prominence

Anterior border of masseter m.

Fig. 9.8 Aesthetic zones of the cheek. (From Sherris DA, Larrabee WF. Principles of Facial Reconstruction: A Subunit Approaoch to Cutaneous Repair. New York, NY: Thieme Medical Publishers; 2009.)

5. The patient doesn't want a skin graft. What do you do?

A moist dressing can be placed on the wound, until final pathology is reported.

6. The final pathology comes back negative. What do you do?

A transposition flap can be used. These include V-Y advancement, bilobed flap (for defects 3–6 cm) or a rhomboid flap.

A V-Y advancement flap is most useful for large defects, or small defects including lid or lateral cheek defects,[2] and rotational flaps are most appropriate for lateral cheek skin because the skin is more densely fixed to underlying structures. Rotational flaps are most useful for defects measuring 3 to 4 cm in the lower preauricular area. Bilobed flaps are most useful for defects 3 to 6 cm (**Table 9.5**).

7. Draw them.

The drawings can be seen in **Fig. 9.9**.

8. You perform a V-Y advancement flap. How do you orient it?

It must be oriented laterally to prevent craniocaudal scar contracture, which can cause a cicatricial ectropion.

9. You plan a transposition flap for a large medial cheek defect, but it doesn't appear that it will reach. What do you do?

Larger rotational flaps, such as the cervicofacial flap or the deltopectoral flap, are useful for larger defects.

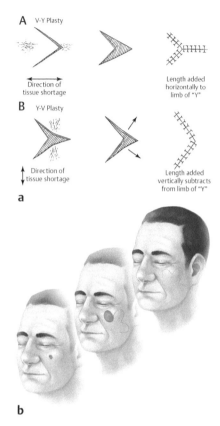

Fig. 9.9 (a) V-Y flap and (b) bilobed flap for cheek reconstruction. (a, From Chen WP. Oculoplastic Surgery: The Essentials. New York, NY: Thieme Medical Publishers; 2001; b, From Gastman, BR. Cutaneous Malignancies. New York, NY: Thieme Medical Publishers; 2017)

Table 9.5 Reconstruction of cheek defects by location and size

Location	Size (cm)	Flap
Lower preauricular	3–4	Rotational
Medial cheek	3–4	Transposition
Any location	3–6	Bilobed flaps
Medial lower eyelid, medial canthus	2–3	V-Y
Buccal cheek	3–6	Rhomboid flap

10. Draw them.
The drawings are shown in **Fig. 9.10**.

11. How much tissue can you get from a deltopectoral flap?
A deltopectoral flap provides tissue for defects of up to 250 cm².

12. The defect is a full-thickness defect of the cheek. What do you do?
A full-thickness defect needs reconstruction of intraoral lining as well as cutaneous coverage. A pectoralis flap is a good pedicled reconstructive option.

13. The defect is thin and involves the corner of the mouth. What do you do?
Complex full-thickness defects that involve multiple functional and aesthetic units are usually best reconstructed with a free flap. The radial forearm free flap is a good option.

14. Draw the harvest.
The drawings can be seen in **Fig. 9.11**.

15. What is your pre-op workup for a radial forearm free flap?
Assuming the patient is otherwise healthy and a nonsmoker, the nondominant arm is preferred as a donor. An Allen test must be performed to confirm that there is filling of the arch through the ulnar artery.

16. You perform a radial forearm free flap. What do you do with the donor site?
A skin graft is the preferred closure method for the donor site. A split-thickness skin graft can be taken from the thigh.

17. You perform a skin graft and there is nontake of the skin graft over flexor carpi radialis (FCR) tendon. What do you do?
In the majority of cases, granulation tissue will form over FCR and the donor site will heal. During the healing process, the tendon is kept moist with a hydrogel and dressing to prevent desiccation. If there is no healing after 3 weeks, consider a bilaminar wound matrix to bridge the gap.

18. During your preoperative workup, you discover the patient has an incomplete palmar arch. What do you do?
In that case, the radial forearm free flap is not an option because of concern of devascularization of the hand. Principles for coverage of cheek defects include reconstruction of layers but thin pliable flaps to allow dynamic movement. Thin fasciocutaneous flaps are most appropriate, and the second choice is an anterolateral thigh (ALT) flap.

19. Draw it.
The drawing can be seen in **Fig. 9.12.**

20. The ALT flap fails. What do you do?
The next choice is a lateral arm flap.

21. Draw it.
The drawing can be seen in **Fig. 9.13.**

Lip Reconstruction

1. How do you assess the lip defect?
The lip defect is assessed by identification of the part of the lip involved, including the philtral columns, philtral dimple, Cupid's bow, white roll, tubercle, commissure, vermillion, and wet and dry roll. Once the involved structures are identified, muscular function is assessed including the pucker response of the orbicularis oris, lip elevation by levator labii superioris centrally and zygomaticus and levator angularis laterally, and lip depression by the depressor labii inferioris. The lower lip is elevated by the mentalis muscle.

2. What are the goals of lip reconstruction?
The goals are replacement of the missing lamellae, including skin and oral lining, preservation or restoration of oral competence,

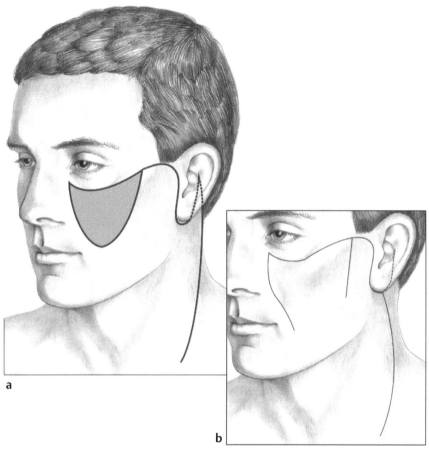

a

b

Fig. 9.10 Carvicofacial flap. (From Sherris DA, Larrabee WF. Principles of Facial Reconstruction: A Subunite Approach to Cutaneous Repair. New York, NY: Thieme Medical Publishers; 2009.)

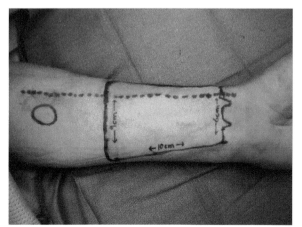

Fig. 9.11   Radial forearm free flap.

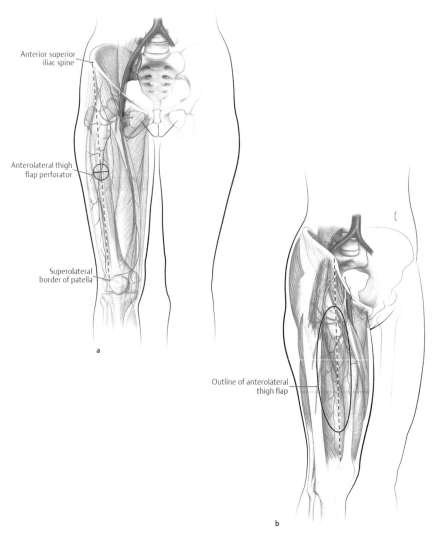

Fig. 9.12 Anterolateral thigh flap. (German G, Levin LS, Sherman R. Reconstructive Surgery of the Hand and Upper Extremity. New York, NY: Thieme Medical Publishers; 2017)

and preservation or restoration of adequate stomal patency (**Table 9.6**).

3. Draw the flaps.
The drawings are shown in **Fig. 9.14.**

4. After reconstruction, the patient is concerned about the color match. What do you do?
After the patient is healed, tattooing on the vermillion is an option for a color match.

5. How can you re-create a beard?
A beard can be re-created by hair transplantation.

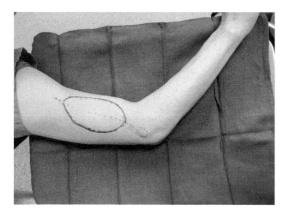

Fig. 9.13 Lateral arm flap design. The dotted circle is over the lateral epicondyle, and the dotted line over the pedicle.

Table 9.6 Reconstruction of lip defects by location and size

	Less than one-third	One-third to two-thirds	Greater than two-thirds	Entire lip
Lower lip defect	Primary closure	Primary closure Abbe's flap Estlander's flap (lateral) Step reconstruction (central)	Karapandzic (central) Webster's Bernard–Burow cheiloplasty	Nasolabial/ mucosal flap Zilinsky's modification of Webster's flap[3] Cervicofacial flap Free flap
Upper lip defect	Primary closure	Abbe's flap Reverse Estlander's flap Cheek advance-ment flap	Microvascular free flap	

Adapted from Rowe NM, Zide B. Lip and oral commissure reconstruction. In: McCarthy JG, Galiano RD, Boutros SG, eds. Current Therapy in Plastic Surgery. Philadelphia, PSaunders Elsevier; 2006.

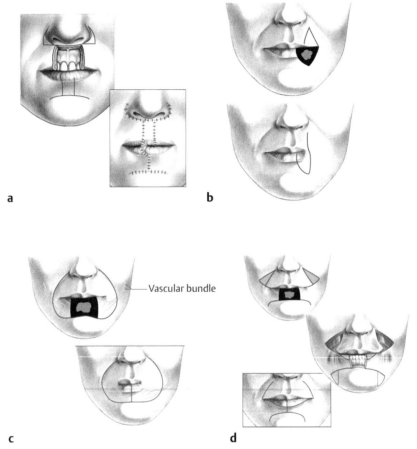

Fig. 9.14   (**a**) Abbe's flap, (**b**) Estlander's flap, (**c**) Karapandzic's flap, and (**d**) Webster's Bernard–Burow cheiloplasty. (From Sherris DA, Larrabee WF. Principles of Facial Reconstruction: A Subunit Approach to Cutaneous Repair. New York, NY: Thieme Medical Publishers; 2009.)

References

1. Alghoul M, Pacella SJ, McClellan WT, Codner MA. Eyelid reconstruction. Plast Reconstr Surg 2013;132(2):288e–302e
2. Heller L, Cole P, Kaufman Y. Cheek reconstruction: current concepts in managing facial soft tissue loss. Semin Plast Surg 2008;22(4):294–305
3. Zilinsky I, Winkler E, Weiss G, Haik J, Tamir J, Orenstein A. Total lower lip reconstruction with innervated muscle-bearing flaps: a modification of the Webster flap. Dermatol Surg 2001;27(7):687–691

10 Aesthetic Surgery for the Aging Face

Abstract

This chapter will review analysis of and surgical options for the aging face, including blepharoplasty, brow lift, and facelift. The reader will be able to analyze the aging face and propose appropriate surgical intervention, and manage postoperative events such as skin flap loss and retrobulbar hematoma.

Keywords: aesthetic surgery, aging face, facelift, facial rejuvenation

Six Key Points

- Facial analysis should proceed from cranial to caudal in thirds
- Pay close attention to the eyes in the aging face.
- Rejuvenation must address volume loss
- Neuropraxias are observed, but visualized nerve injuries are repaired.
- Skin slough is managed conservatively.
- Initial masnagement of any outcome that can be attributed to scarring is scar massage and observation.

Questions

Case 1

A 64-year-old woman presents for rejuvenation of the face.

1. What do you see?
The face is evaluated for overall skin quality, sun damage, and presence of rhytids. It is then evaluated from cranial to caudal. The forehead is evaluated for rhytids as well as relative length and location of the hairline, which can have implications for forehead shortening and incision placement for a brow lift. The brow is noted for its position, and any brow ptosis is noted. The eyes are evaluated for dermatochalasis and ptosis, as well as any indicators of eyelid disease or general health from the sclera, such as diffusely injected sclera, or scleral icterus. The position and tone of the lower lids is noted, as well as the vector of the eye. The nasolabial folds are noted, and their relative prominence, as are perioral rhytids and the presence of marionette lines. Overall atrophy of facial soft tissue is noted.

2. What do you offer the patient?
A facelift is the most appropriate intervention to address mid- and lower face descent. I would offer a superficial musculoaponeurotic system (SMAS) plication facelift. If the patient also has brow and eyelid issues, it is offered as a staged approach—first the brow and the eyelids, then the face and neck, and finally laser resurfacing if indicated.

3. Explain why an SMAS plication is offered and draw your incision.
See **Fig. 10.1** for incisions. The incision goes from the temporal hairline to a pretragal incision, wrapping around the earlobe to extend posteriorly into the hairline. There are several techniques for a facelift, including a skin-only facelift, in which the SMAS layer is not addressed, an SMAS-ectomy, in which redundant muscle is removed, and other variations. A skin-only facelift will

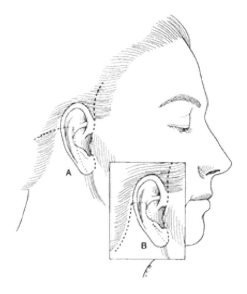

Fig. 10.1 Incision placement for a facelift. SMAS, superficial musculoaponeurotic system. From Wobig JL, Dailey RA. Oculofacial Plastic Surgery: Face, Lacrimal System, and Orbit. New York, NY: Thieme Medical Publishers; 2004.

not address the muscle and the differential vectors of descent. Because of the path of the facial nerve branches, which lie on the sub-SMAS level, resecting SMAS not only uses the volume of the SMAS layer, but also runs the risk of injuring the facial nerve branches. An SMAS plication will preserve volume while avoiding facial nerve branches. The SMAS plication is performed over the zygoma, and the zygomatic retaining ligaments and mandibular retaining ligaments must be released to reposition the skin over the plicated SMAS.

4. What do you do about the neck?

A separate, approximately 4 cm, submental incision is used. This incision is placed posterior to the submental crease, between the mentum and hyoid, because placement within the submental crease can create a persistent double chin deformity. This separate incision allows for access to the anterior neck. If there is platysmal banding, the dissection proceeds in the intermediate plane of the neck. Facelift scissors are used to create skin flaps. Excess fat can be directly excised, as long as at least 5 mm of fat is left

on the skin. The platysma muscle is exposed to the boundaries of thyroid cartilage subplatysmal fat, anterior bellies of the digastric muscles, and submandibular glands. In this dissection, there is release of the submental retaining ligaments. The anterior bellies of the digastric muscles can be excised if needed, or they can be plicated, followed by platysmal plication.[1] The space is irrigated, and the submental incision is closed last, after hemostasis has been obtained under the facelift flaps.

5. Postoperatively, she calls to report that she has swelling on the left side of her face. What do you do?

The first step is to bring her in to evaluate her and exclude a hematoma, which can occur approximately 4% of the time. Even if there are drains in place and a compression dressing, a hematoma can occur. Because a hematoma can affect the viability of the skin flaps, it is important to identify it and drain it. If she has a hematoma on examination, plan operative intervention by obtaining informed consent and alerting the operating room staff. The hematoma is evacuated surgically and potential causes of bleeding are identified. Once hemostasis has been confirmed, the incisions are reclosed.

6. What other things would you do?

Risk factors for hematoma are high blood pressure, medications or herbal supplements that decrease clotting ability, and traumatic events such as shear injury, which may disrupt a clot. Thus, I would ensure that she is normotensive, that, she is not taking any medication that may decrease clotting ability, and that drains and compression dressing are replaced. If the hematoma is a late presentation, and there is suspicion that it has liquefied, which can happen in about a week, the hematoma can be aspirated in the office.

7. She complains of decreased movement of her lower lip. What do you do?

Facial nerve injuries can happen in a face lift and are part of the informed consent process. Initially, I would wait because it may represent a neuropraxia, and I would counsel her that it may recover on its own. Use of a sub-SMAS dissection plane increases the risk of a nerve injury fourfold. If a nerve injury is identified intraoperatively, it should be repaired in the operating room.

8. How do you repair the nerve?

The repair is done with microsurgical instruments, and with microscopic magnification. The two ends of the nerve are identified. The branch can be confirmed with a nerve stimulator, which will work up to approximately 72 hours after surgery, and an epineural repair is performed with 8–0 or 9–0 nylon.

9. She comes back a week later and she has skin slough. What do you do?

It is managed conservatively with ointment such as Bacitracin. Silver sulfadiazine is avoided because it can cause skin

darkening. The area is allowed to heal by secondary intention.

10. It is possible to excise that area and do a small rotational flap, which she hopes will get her healed sooner.

Despite pressure from the patient, it is still appropriate to manage it conservatively.

Case 2

A 67-year-old woman presents for eyelid rejuvenation.

1. What do you see?

The eyes are assessed beginning at the brows. It is important to note whether the brow is in good position, which is at the supraorbital rim in men and slightly above it in women, and to note whether it is in place because of compensatory frontalis contraction, which may indicate underlying brow ptosis.

Eyelids should be assessed for excess skin as well as blepharoptosis, which is measured by the marginal reflex distance (**Fig. 10.2**). The elasticity of the lower lid should be measured by the snap-back test and the pinch test (**Table 10.1**).

In addition, Bell's phenomenon should be assessed.

A history should include assessment for dry eyes and the use of eye drops, and physical examination may include Schirmer's test (**Table 10.2**).

2. How is Schirmer's test performed?

As in **Table 10.1**, a paper strip is placed in the inferior fornix for 5 minutes. The distance that a tear film has traveled is measured on the strip. Normal is greater than 15 mm. Postoperatively, tear flow can be disrupted, and dry eyes can be exacerbated.

3. What do you offer the patient?

In a patient with brow ptosis, dermatochalasis, and lower lid laxity and redundancy, a brow lift and upper and lower blepharoplasty are offered.

4. Describe your brow lift.

An endoscopic brow lift is offered for patients without significant forehead elongation and with mild forehead rhytids. The procedure is done under monitored anesthesia care or under general anesthesia. The port sites are marked in horizontal positions at the midline, 0.5 cm posterior to the hairline, and laterally in the temple area 7 and 10 cm from the midline and approximately 2 cm posterior to the hairline. The forehead is injected with local anesthetic with epinephrine 1:100,000 and the

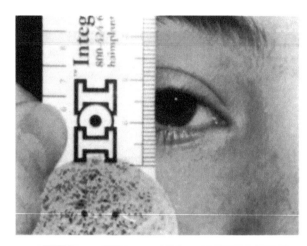

Fig. 10.2 Marginal reflex distance (MRD). The palpebral fissure is the distance between the upper and lower lid margins in primary gaze. Normal height is 7 to 10 mm in males and 8 to 12 mm in females. The patient should be examined closely for ptosis if the fissure distance is less than 10 mm. Normal MRD1 is 4 to 4.5 mm. Mild ptosis is associated with an MRD1 of 2 mm, moderate ptosis is associated with an MRD1 of 1 mm, and severe ptosis is less than 0 mm. (From Wobig JL, Dailey RA. Oculofacial Plastic Surgery: Face, Lacrimal System, and Orbit. New York, NY: Thieme Medical Publishers; 2004.)

Table 10.1 Grading of snap-back test and pinch test

	Time to return to position	**Grade**
Snap-back test	Immediately on release, fraction of second	0
	2–3 s	I
	4–5 s	II
	> 5 s, returns with blinking	III
Margin limbal distance	Does not return to position	IV
Pinch test	**Distance moved medially**	**Grade**
Medial movement of lateral canthus with pinch	2–4 mm	I
	4–6 mm	II
	> 6 mm	III
	No spontaneous return to baseline	IV

Table 10.2 Eyelid tests to perform prior to eyelid surgery

Eyelid tests

Name	Description	Normal	Notes
Vertical fissure height	Distance between upper and lower lids at level of pupil in forward gaze	10 mm vertical, 30 mm horizontal	
Levator function, Berke's method	With brow immobile, patient looks from extreme downgaze to upgaze and the millimeter movement of the upper lid is measured	> 15 mm. Good: 12–14 mm; fair: 5–11mm; poor: < 4 mm	
MRD1	Distance from light reflex to upper lid margin	4–4.5 mm	
MRD2	Distance from light reflex to lower lid	4.5–5.5 mm	
Margin limbal distance	Distance from central lower lid to central upper lid on extreme upgaze		
MRD3	Distance from light reflex to central upper lid margin in extreme upgaze		
Bell's phenomenon	Open lids while patient is tightly closing eyes; eyes should be in upgaze		Risk of exposure keratopathy if not present
Hering's law	Equal innervation to eyelids		
Mueller's muscle function	10% phenylephrine is applied to the eye; if ptosis corrects, resection of Mueller's muscle may correct the ptosis		
Schirmer's test	Paper strip placed in inferior fornix for five minutes	> 15 mm. Mild: 9–14 mm; moderate: 4–8 mm; severe: < 4 mm	

Abbreviation: MRD marginal reflex distance.

incision site in the hair-bearing regions are injected with local anesthetic with epinephrine 1:200,000. The lateral-most port site is incised with a knife, and the most lateral incision is continued to the deep temporal fascia, which is then further exposed with a baby Metzenbaum scissors. The access port is placed to expose the plane between the superficial and deep temporal fascia. A periosteal elevator is used to sweep toward the more medial incision, which is medial to deep temporal fascia and at the level of periosteum, which is incised such that the plane of dissection is subperiosteal. The midline incision is made after the lateral incisions are made and the sites connected. A 30-degree 4-mm endoscope is placed in the lateral-most incision. A periosteal elevator is used to dissect in the subperiosteal plane to the supraorbital rim, and proceeds from lateral to medial. The supraorbital and supratrochlear nerves are identified, and a grasper is used to remove the corrugator muscle. The procedure is repeated on the opposite side, and fat grafts are taken from a rent in the deep temporal fascia cephalad to the medial aspect of the zygomatic arch. Hemostasis is obtained. A fascial suspension suture is placed through the superficial temporal fascia of the lateral-most incision, and secured to the posterior aspect of the incision. If needed, a second suspension suture is placed through the more medial incision, and passed through a bone tunnel made by a 1.1-mm burr with entrances 4 mm apart and 4 mm deep. Endotine can also be used at this point for additional fixation. A small drain is placed, and the incisions are closed in layers.

RATIONALE: An endoscopic brow lift is the best choice for patients with a normal forehead length, mild rhytids, and brow ptosis. There are other options besides an endoscopic brow lift for forehead rejuvenation, depending on the specific physical examination findings. Patients with rhytids who do not have significant brow ptosis can have *botulinum toxin A, fillers*, or *fat injections*. Patients who have rhytids associated with the corrugator muscle alone can undergo a *transpalpebral corrugator resection*, which can be combined with a blepharoplasty and is appropriate for patients with receding hairlines, in particular male patients. For patients with elongated foreheads or receding foreheads and deep wrinkles, the best choices are a subcutaneous forehead rhytidectomy or a *scalp advancement.*

5. After surgery, the patient reports forehead dimpling and notes that she believes she looks surprised all the time. Why did that happen?

The most likely reason for dimpling is irregular corrugator resection, a common cause of an unfavorable result. The surprised look is most often caused by over-release of the medial soft tissue and overcorrection of eyebrow position.[2]

6. When do you offer a canthopexy?

A canthopexy is offered to avoid lid malposition. It is performed if there is lid laxity of the lower lid. It must be considered very carefully in patients with a negative vector (**Fig. 10.3**).

7. Postoperatively, she comes back and the left canthus appears higher than the right. What do you do?

Initially postoperatively, the placement is slightly higher. It is expected to settle, and the initial steps are scar massage and observation.

8. She develops an ectropion. What do you do?

Initially, the treatment is scar massage and LACRI-LUBE for corneal protection. If it persists, the eyelid must be assessed systematically by lamella to determine the etiology of the ectropion.

Ectropion can be considered by pathology and by anatomy.

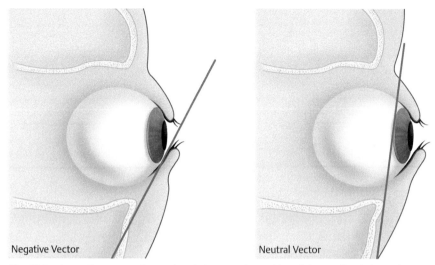

Fig. 10.3   A negative vector refers to the relative posterior position of the maxilla relative to the globe. A canthopexy in the context of a negative vector increases the risk of scleral show as the lower lid is pulled inferiorly on the globe.

References

1. Mejia JD, Nahai FR, Nahai F, Momoh AO. Isolated management of the aging neck. Semin Plast Surg 2009;23(4):264–273

2. Guyuron B. Endoscopic forehead rejuvenation: I. Limitations, flaws, and rewards. Plast Reconstr Surg 2006;117(4):1121–1133, discussion 1134–1136

11 Facial Trauma

Abstract

This chapter will review facial trauma, and specifically facial fractures including mandible fractures, orbital fractures, zygoma fractures, and panfacial fractures. The reader will be able to analyze plain films and CT scans of these fractures and propose surgical plans, as well as describe incisions and explain management of intraoperative and postoperative events and poor outcomes.

Keywords: facial trauma, panfacial fractures, zygoma fractures

Six Key Points

- Bilateral condylar neck fractures have anterior open bites; reapply maxillo-mandibular fixation if you see anterior open bite after removal.
- Always fix stable to unstable ("top to bottom," "lateral to medial").
- Complex fractures have discrete sequences of fixation.
- Enophthalmos can be caused by increased bony orbit or by loss of soft tissue.
- Diplopia can be caused by inadequate fixation or by muscle fibrosis.
- Restoring buttresses is necessary.

Overview

Mandible Fractures

Mandible fractures affect the symphysis, parasymphysis, body, angle, ramus, subcondyle, and condyle. Because of the curvature of the mandible, it is common to have fracture in two places; and identification of one fracture should trigger examination for another fracture. Maxillo-mandibular fixation (MMF) will treat all mandible fractures provided occlusion has been set; open reduction and internal fixation, however, are preferred for those fractures that are amenable to it because of earlier return to function. The surgical sequence of mandible fracture fixation is as follows: arch bar placement, fracture exposure, occlusal and bone reduction, checking condyles are in glenoid fossae, rigid fixation, release intermaxillary fixation (IMF) and check occlusion, closure, and elastic application if needed.

Naso-orbitoethmoid Fractures

The first step of naso-orbitoethmoid (NOE) fracture repair is identifying the type of fracture (type 1, 2, or 3). Associated injuries are assessed. The repair will be determined by the type of fracture; while all require some sort of operative fixation, the reconstruction of the medial canthal ligament (MCL) will depend on whether the MCL remains attached to bone. The repair of NOE fractures consists, in general, of eight discrete steps: surgical exposure, identification of the medial canthal tendon, reduction and reconstruction of the medial orbital rim, reconstruction of the medial orbital wall, transnasal canthopexy, reduction of septal fractures, nasal dorsum reconstruction, and soft-tissue reconstruction.[1]

Frontal Sinus Fractures

The clinical question in frontal sinus fractures is whether the frontonasal ducts are damaged. A frontal sinus fracture is, for that reason, potentially dangerous. If there is no nasofrontal outflow injury, the anterior table can be repaired. If there is nasofrontal outflow injury with obstruction, the sinus must be cranialized or obliterated (**Fig. 11.1**). On the films, air in the sinus is an indication that the sinus is draining. The anterior wall can be reconstructed with small plates, or with mesh if there is comminution. The sinus is obliterated by burring the bone, and filling it with bone and fibrin glue.

If there is a displaced fracture of the posterior wall, there will be air-fluid levels and pneumocephalus, and neurosurgery must be involved. In cases of anterior and posterior wall injuries, as well as floor injuries, the sequence of repair is as follows: remove the posterior wall and dural repair (by neurosurgery), reconstruct the anterior wall, and put bone graft (with or without a flap) to the floor.

Zygomaticomaxillary Complex Fractures

Zygomaticomaxillary complex (ZMC) fractures are associated with orbital floor injury, and if the zygoma undergoes reduction and an orbital floor fracture becomes manifest, enophthalmos can ensue. Thus, the risk of enophthalmos because of an increased orbital volume is an indication for exploration. One should keep in mind that exposure of the inferior orbit has risk of scleral show.[2] The sequence of steps is to reduce the lateral buttress, with the infraorbital rim if needed. If it is stable, no fixation may be necessary. If it is unstable, plate the ZM buttress with a 1.7-mm plate. If the reduction is adequate but continues to be unstable, the zygomaticofrontal (ZF) suture should be plated with a 1.2-mm plate. If after plating of the ZM buttress the reduction is inadequate and unstable, the ZF suture and lateral orbital wall should be exposed and plated. If after exposure and plating of the ZM buttress and the ZF suture there is still inadequate reduction and

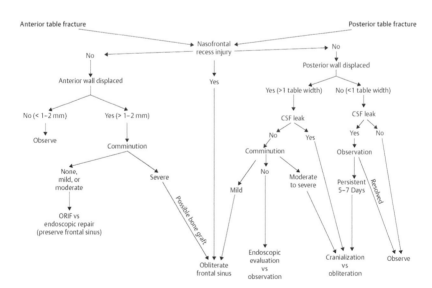

Fig. 11.1 Frontal sinus fracture algorithm.

instability, the infraorbital rim should be exposed, reduced, and plated with a 1.7-mm plate (**Fig. 11.2**).

Orbital Fractures

Orbital fractures are significant because there is a precise balance between the bony orbit and the contents. The antrum and ethmoid are convex, and with fracture the contour becomes concave. Enophthalmos results from mismatch of the bony orbit and the contents—the concave contour causes an increase in the size (and thus, volume) of the bony orbit, and the contents settle into that concavity. Indications for surgical intervention of orbital fractures are the following: trapdoor fracture causing entrapment of muscles and restriction of ocular movement, potential for volume changes, or persistent diplopia. While postoperative enophthalmos should always trigger evaluation to ensure that there has been adequate reduction of the bony orbit, it is important to remember and counsel patients that the trauma itself can cause atrophy of the soft tissues, which can lead to enophthalmos (**Table 11.1**).

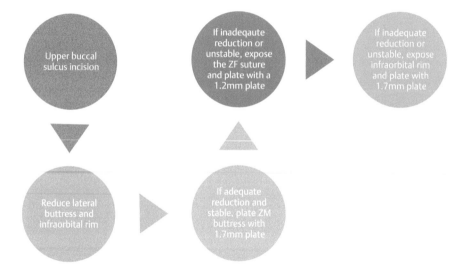

Fig. 11.2 Zygomatic complex fracture fixation sequence. (Adapted from Ricketts S, Gill HS, Fialkov JA, Matic DB, Antonyshyn OM. Facial fractures. Plast Reconstr Surg 2016;137(2):424e–444e)

Table 11.1 Timing of orbital surgery

Timing of orbital surgery	Indication
Acute	Trapdoor
Early repair	Potential for volume change enophthalmos
Early exploration	Persistent diplopia, acute enophthalmos, large defect in the critical bulge

Panfacial Fractures

Panfacial fractures are simply a combination of facial fractures. Each fracture pattern is repaired according to its principles, and the reconstructive goals are restoration of function, facial width, and facial height. Reconstruction follows stability; usually, the most cranial fracture is repaired, and then the sequence runs caudally. Assessment and treatment of panfacial fractures requires determination of facial width, using the zygoma or lateral orbital wall as a guide, and facial height, using the mandible as a guide (or, if the mandible is not available, the maxillary buttresses). Panfacial fracture repair includes five steps (**Fig. 11.3**).

Questions

Case 1

Comminuted ZMC fracture, inferior orbital fracture, alveolar fracture and high subcondylar fracture

1. What would you do?

Assuming he or she has been cleared for other injury and c-spine trauma, proceed with operative repair.
RATIONALE: About 10% of facial trauma is associated with c-spine injury.

2. How do you approach the CT scan?

First, assess the soft-tissue envelope for air and swelling. Evaluate the bones for fractures, and assess the zygomatic arch, the position of the condylar heads, the width of the maxilla (which is a proxy for midface width), and the mandible.

3. What are your reconstructive aims?

Restoring function (such as jaw opening, or decreasing diplopia), and restoring facial projections, facial height, and facial width.

4. How do you approach it?

Multiple incisions, including a lateral brow incision and a lateral transconjunctival incision (**Table 11.2**).

5. How do you use the buttresses?

The buttresses provide support, and there are four anterior buttresses and two posterior buttresses. The midface buttresses are affected by occlusion, but these relationships are dynamic.

6. What is the approach?

With a true panfacial fracture, the first step is to identify the width. One starts at the skull base and moves caudally. If there is a disruption of the frontozygomatic suture, one uses a temporary wire at the articulation of the frontozygomatic suture. One then plates the posterior arch, and then the wire is removed and the frontozygomatic suture is plated. The NOE fracture is then plated, and then occlusion is addressed. After occlusion has been addressed, the maxillary buttresses are plated, and gaps in the buttresses are replaced with bone grafts.

7. What are the considerations if there is a sagittal palatal fracture and a condylar neck fracture?

One must be very aware of occlusion because one must plate the palate before the patient is put in occlusion.

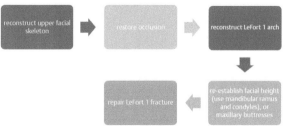

Fig. 11.3 Five steps of panfacial fractures (Adapted from Ricketts S, Gill HS, Fialkov JA, Matic DB, Antonyshyn OM. Facial fractures. Plast Reconstr Surg 2016;137(2):424e–444e)

Table 11.2   Incision choice for facial fractures

Incision	Subtype	Facial skeleton then can be accessed	Advantages	Disadvantages
Coronal		Upper facial skeletal and midface skeleton, including zygomatic arch	Excellent exposure	Large incision, resuspension of soft tissues is needed, risk of damage to temporal branch of facial nerve
Lower eyelid		Inferior orbit	Good access to inferior rim	Limited medial wall access, ectropion risk
Transconjunctival	Preseptal	Inferior orbit	Can access inferior orbital rim better than retroseptal	
	Retroseptal	Inferior orbit	Access to medial orbital wall, lower risk of lid shortening	Risk of entropion from lower lid retractor release, limited access to inferior orbital rim
Upper eyelid		Lateral orbit	Well-hidden scar	Limited exposure
Maxillary vestibular		Midfacial skeleton, from zygomatic arch to infraorbital rim to frontal process of the maxilla	Intraoral incision, low risk of damage to facial nerve if in subperiosteal plane	Often needs another incision if infraorbital rim exposure is needed
Mandibular vestibular		Mandible (although condylar and subcondylar access less exposed	Intraoral incision	Risk of witch's chin if mentalis muscle not resuspended
Submandibular	Risdon	Mandibular body and ramus	Exposure of body angle and ramus	Risk of damage to marginal mandibular nerve
Retromandibular		Mandibular ramus	Exposure of condylar neck/ head, or ramus itself	Risk of damage to parotid gland and facial nerve (marginal mandibular branch)
Rhytidectomy		Mandibular ramus, condyle, condylar neck	Similar to retromandibular approach but hidden scar	Risk of injury to greater auricular nerve, added time for closure
Preauricular		Access to the condyle	Well-hidden scar and excellent exposure of condyle	Risk of injury to facial nerve

Table 11.3   Manson's classification

Type	Features	Treatment
1	Single central fragment	Reduction, plating, wiring if central canthal
2	Comminution of central fragment	Same as type 1
3	Disruption of medial canthal tendon	Open transnasal canthoplasty, posterosuperior vector

Source: Adapted from Lakin GE. Plastic Surgery Review: A Study Guide for the In-Service, Written Board, and Maintenance of Certification Exams. New York, NY: Thieme Medical Publishers; 2015.

8. How do you classify NOE fractures?
Manson's classification (**Table 11.3**).

Craniofacial Fractures

1. Do you repair craniofacial fractures with neurosurgery or after neurosurgery?
Perform the repair at the same time as neurosurgery, with monitoring of intracranial pressure (ICP).
RATIONALE: Repair is safe if ICP is less than 15 mm Hg. A combined repair will allow for harvest of cranial bone grafts, if needed. A staged repair can run the risk of disrupting the dural repair, and a decreased ability for a sea of the cranial cavity and frontal sinus.

2. How do you perform the repair?
With monitoring of ICP with neurosurgery, facial projection and width is reestablished by stabilizing the frontal bar, then the lateral orbits, and then the zygomatic arch.

3. How would you make your surgical approach?
Through multiple incisions: lateral brow, transconjunctival with lateral canthotomy, buccal sulcus.

4. Once everything is exposed, what do you do?
Approach from stable to unstable, usually in a craniocaudal direction, and from lateral to medial: addressing the "outer frame" (zygomatic arch, zygoma, and frontal bar), followed by the "inner frame" (NOE complex). The mandible is a guide for width, lip–tooth relationship for midface height, and the lateral orbital wall is a guide for ZMC reduction. With the patient in MMF, the orbital floor and medial and lateral buttresses should be plated.

5. For subcondylar fractures, how long do you leave the patient in MMF?
The patient is kept in MMF for 2 weeks, but arch bars are kept in place after 2 weeks.

6. You release MMF and there is still an anterior open bite. What do you do?
Scan to reassess. If the reduction is okay, you can place the patient in guiding elastics.

7. You do that for 2 weeks and there is still an anterior open bite. What do you do?
If there has not been a recent scan, one would consider a CT scan to assess for lost reduction or for hardware failure or infection.

8. Now the patient has diplopia. What do you do?
Diplopia should be evaluated with a forced duction test to exclude entrapment. Enophthalmos should also be excluded as a causative factor. In some cases, persistent diplopia is because of fibrosis and scarring of the extraocular muscles.

9. Now the patient has enophthalmos. What happened?
Enophthalmos is caused by inadequate reduction, or loss of soft tissue. Soft-tissue loss can be because of fat atrophy from the injury itself.

Case 2

A 35 y/o female patient presents to the ER after a motor vehicle crash with a complex panfacial fracture with an NOE frature, frontal sinus fracture, and palatal fracture.

1. What do you do?
Assess for concomitant c-spine injury.

2. What is your indication for bone grafting?
Primary bone grafting is indicated for a bony gap.

RATIONALE: Delayed bone grafting becomes difficult because of soft-tissue contraction and scarring, loss of pliability, and a scarred bone graft bed. A long graft can be taken from the rib, and a calvarial bone graft can be taken from the posterior cranium.

3. How would you approach the NOE fracture?
The exposure would include a coronal incision with an upper buccal sulcus incision and a lower lid incision.

Case 3

A 20-year-old male with facial deformity several weeks after a motor vehicle crash. Physical examination reveals an impacted NOE segment with a depressed frontal sinus. CT scan imaging demonstrates fractured anterior and posterior tables of the frontal sinus and an orbital floor defect.

1. What do you do?
After assessing for concomitant injuries and ruling out life-threatening injuries, the patient is consented for operative reduction. The reconstructive goals are to protect the cranial contents, re-create a normal forehead contour, preserve frontonasal duct function if possible, and to prevent a mucocele, and to reduce the orbital floor fracture to prevent enophthalmos. If the posterior table is mildly communited, sinus obliteration is an option. If there is severe comminution, cranialization is indicated. The approach includes wide exposure with coronal incisions and orbital incisions. During the exposure, a pericranial flap is preserved for nasofrontal duct obliteration.

Neurosurgery would be involved to help perform the craniotomy, to remove the posterior table, and to cranialize the sinus. Mucosa is removed from the sinus walls, and the ducts are obliterated with nonvascularized temporalis fascia and calvarial bone graft. An NOE segment posterior to the lacrimal fossa is osteotomized, and the intercanthal distance is set within the normal range (~ 30–31 mm). The orbital floor is repaired with either a MEDPOR implant or a plate, and secured to the orbital rim.

References

1. Ellis E III. Sequencing treatment for naso-orbito-ethmoid fractures. J Oral Maxillofac Surg 1993;51(5):543–558
2. Ricketts S, Gill HS, Fialkov JA, Matic DB, Antonyshyn OM. Facial fractures. Plast Reconstr Surg 2016;137(2):424e–444e

12 Breast Reconstruction

Abstract

This chapter will review surgical options for breast reconstruction including expander-based and autologous reconstructions, and the indications and limitations of each, as well as the role of radiation. The reader will be able to manage the mastectomy site and the irradiated bed for purposes of reconstruction, and will be able to create step-wise surgical reconstructive plans and manage complications.

Keywords: breast reconstruction, tissue expansion, nipple reconstruction

Six Key Points

- Reconstruction can be either implant based or autologous.
- Implant reconstruction in irradiated beds is associated with higher complication rates.
- Cancer can be upstaged on final pathology, which must be considered when performing an immediate reconstruction.
- Tissue expanders can be overfilled.
- Food and Drug Administration (FDA) recommends MRI screening for silent ruptures 3 years after placement of silicone implants, and every 2 years after that.
- Latissimus flaps can be more reliable in patients with a BMI > 35.

Questions

Case 1

A 45-year-old female presents for unilateral breast reconstruction, without radiation (**Fig. 12.1**).

1. The patient presents prior to mastectomy to discuss reconstructive options. What do you tell her?

First, confirm the oncologic plan and whether postoperative radiation is needed. A targeted history should be performed looking specifically for intrinsic (such as bleeding or thrombotic disorders) and extrinsic factors (such as smoking) as they may affect the reconstructive options. Her goals for reconstruction should be identified, including whether she would prefer implant-based reconstruction or autologous reconstruction.

2. Would you offer her immediate reconstruction?

"Immediate" reconstruction can refer to either a reconstructive procedure at the time of mastectomy or a definitive reconstruction at the time of mastectomy. There are two reasons to stage reconstruction with a tissue expander first, then definitive reconstruction. This first is to confirm the oncologic status. The second reason is to confirm that the mastectomy flaps are viable, and to allow for debridement of the mastectomy flaps if they are not.

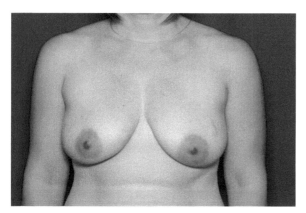

Fig. 12.1 A patient presents for breast reconstruction.

RATIONALE: Oncologic status must be confirmed, because the diagnosis can change on final pathology. Core biopsy can be inaccurate—approximately 18% of specimens with a core needle biopsy diagnosis of atypical ductal hyperplasia will be upstaged to either ductal carcinoma in situ (DCIS) or invasive cancer, and approximately 20% of DCIS specimens will be upstaged to invasive cancer, depending on associated clinical and histological characteristics.[1–5] A change in final pathology may result in the need for further surgical intervention.

3. How do you determine what expander to use?

The expander size is determined by the base width. This can be determined by the width of the breast, but with a large breast, the width can extend laterally on the chest wall and the expander itself can have the lateral aspect extending to the axilla. Once a subpectoral pocket is created, the width of the pocket can be measured with a ruler, and the implant can be sized.

4. How do you cover the implant?

The implant can be either entirely submuscular or partially submuscular. In an entirely submuscular implant, the pectoralis muscle fibers remain attached to the rib caudally, and serratus muscle and fascia is elevated laterally and sewn to the lateral edge of pectoralis major muscle. In a partially submuscular implant, the pectoralis muscle fibers are detached from their rib attachments, and an acellular dermal matrix sling is placed.

5. How do you decide whether to use a complete submuscular placement or a subpectoral pocket?

A complete submuscular placement provides two distinct advantages: it reduces the risk of infection and the risk of lateral displacement of the implant. The limitations of the approach are that the expander may be positioned more cephalad than with a subpectoral pocket.

A subpectoral pocket is created when the caudal attachments of the pectoralis major muscle to the ribs are released. The expander has muscular coverage superiorly and medially. Use of a "sling," or suturing acellular dermal matrix to the edge of pectoralis muscle, allows some coverage of the implant inferiorly and prevents caudal displacement of the implant. The advantage of this approach is that the implant can be positioned caudally near the intermaxillary fixation (IMF) and has less of a tendency for cephalad displacement, and allows more significant lower pole expansion, but there is a higher risk of expander exposure and seroma.

A complete submuscular placement is used for the following indications: questionably viable skin flaps or thin skin flaps (such as in very thin individuals).

6. What are the risks of decellularized dermal matrix?

There is a higher risk of seroma with Alloderm™ (Life-Cell, Branchburg, NJ)[6] and there is the risk of "red breast syndrome".[7] Red breast syndrome is a nonpainful erythema of the skin overlying acellular dermal matrix, not associated with warmth of the skin. Because it is acellular, there is minimal risk of rejection, and it allows from vascular ingrowth.[8]

7. Do you overfill the expander?

Expanders are typically overfilled by approximately 20%. After the overexpansion, the pocket is allowed to mature for at least 1 month, although some wait longer.

8. She is expanded and you place an implant. How do you decide whether to use a saline or silicone implant?

The risks and benefits of saline versus silicone implants are reviewed with the patient. Silicone implants have "silent ruptures" in which the shell ruptures are undetected on physical examination, and unnoticed by the patient, as opposed to saline, which gets resorbed by the body. Food and Drug Administration (FDA) recommendations are for silicone implants to be monitored by MRI for silent rupture 3 years after placement, and every 2 years after that.

RATIONALE: In the overwhelming majority of cases, the decision to use a silicone or a saline implant is made by the patient, and the plastic surgeon's role is to provide information about the risks and benefits of saline or silicone implants. It is important to note for young patients with breast cancer that while silicone implants are FDA approved for reconstructive purposes in any age, they are approved for women age 22 years and older for cosmetic purposes.

9. After reconstruction, she desires nipple areolar complex reconstruction. What are the options?

There are over 15 described nipple reconstruction methods. Of these, the most popular are the skate flaps, the star flap, and the C-V flap.

10. Draw it.

The drawings can be seen in **Fig. 12.2**.

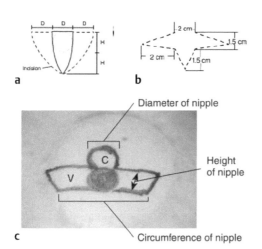

a

b

c

Fig. 12.2 (**a**) The skate flap, (**b**) star flap, and (**c**) C-V flap. (Adapted from Janis JE. Essentials of Plastic Surgery. 2nd ed. New York, NY: Thieme Medical Publishers; 2014.)

Diameter of nipple

Height of nipple

Circumference of nipple

11. After your surgery, she is discovered to be a carrier of the BRCA mutation. What do you do now?

She may want to proceed with a prophylactic mastectomy on the contralateral side. In that case, reconstruction is performed based on the previous reconstruction. If she has had an implant reconstruction, it can be matched. If she has had an abdominally based reconstruction, she will need another form of reconstruction, and may need additional procedures for size matching.

Case 2

A 45-year-old woman presents for bilateral breast reconstruction, with planned radiation on the left.

1. What do you offer the patient?

The first step is to obtain a thorough history of the patient and determine risk factors for wound healing, such as smoking history, and risk factors for clotting disorders. A history of abdominal surgeries should also be obtained.

With planned radiation, the first step is placement of tissue expanders at the time of mastectomy (see above).

2. What is your expansion protocol?

The tissue expanders are allowed to heal for approximately 1 month, and then expansion is started. Some radiation oncologists prefer minimal expansion on the left side prior to expansion because of the impact on the heart.[9]

3. What do you offer the patient?

After the patient has completed radiation, if additional expansion needs to be performed, it is performed 6 months after radiation to allow the tissues to stabilize. Expansion proceeds slowly and as tolerated by the patient. Once the

expander is fully expanded, after 1 month reconstruction of the breast mound is offered. In the case of radiation, assuming the BMI is less than 35, the patient may be a candidate for a deep inferior epigastric perforator free flap. In patients with BMI greater than 35, a latissimus flap is more reliable.

References

1. Dillon MF, Quinn CM, McDermott EW, O'Doherty A, O'Higgins N, Hill AD. Diagnostic accuracy of core biopsy for ductal carcinoma in situ and its implications for surgical practice. J Clin Pathol 2006;59(7):740–743

2. Kurniawan ED, Rose A, Mou A, et al. Risk factors for invasive breast cancer when core needle biopsy shows ductal carcinoma in situ. Arch Surg 2010;145(11):1098–1104

3. Mandell J. Breast imaging. In: Core Radiology: A Visual Approach to Diagnostic Imaging. Cambridge: Cambridge University Press; 2013:593

4. Moran CJ, Kell MR, Flanagan FL, Kennedy M, Gorey TF, Kerin MJ. Role of sentinel lymph node biopsy in high-risk ductal carcinoma in situ patients. Am J Surg 2007;194(2):172–175

5. Szynglarewicz B, Kasprzak P, Halon A, Matkowski R. Preoperatively diagnosed ductal cancers in situ of the breast presenting as even small masses are of high risk for the invasive cancer foci in postoperative specimen. World J Surg Oncol 2015;13:218

6. Ganske I, Hoyler M, Fox SE, Morris DJ, Lin SJ, Slavin SA. Delayed hypersensitivity reaction to acellular dermal matrix in breast reconstruction: the red breast syndrome? Ann Plast Surg 2014;73 (suppl 2):S139–S14

7. Menon NG, Rodriguez ED, Byrnes CK, Girotto JA, Goldberg NH, Silverman RP.

Revascularization of human acellular dermis in full-thickness abdominal wall reconstruction in the rabbit model. Ann Plast Surg 2003;50(5):523–52

8. Ho G, Nguyen TJ, Shahabi A, Hwang BH, Chan LS, Wong AK. A systematic review and meta-analysis of complications associated with acellular dermal matrix-assisted breast reconstruction. Ann Plast Surg 2012;68(4):346–356

9. Motwani SB, Strom EA, Schechter NR, et al. The impact of immediate breast reconstruction on the technical delivery of postmastectomy radiotherapy. Int J Radiat Oncol Biol Phys 2006;66(1):76–82

13 Elective Breast Surgery

Abstract

This chapter will review elective breast surgery, including breast reduction, augmentation, and mastopexy. The reader will be able to manage the large breast, the small breast, and assess and address complications.

Keywords: macromastia, micromastia, reduction mammoplasty, breast reduction

Six Key Points

- Breast surgery should take into consideration the skin envelope and the breast parenchyma, and the footprint of the breast.
- The nipple-areolar complex can be assessed for viability intraoperatively with fluorescein.
- Breast implants should be chosen based on the base width of the patient's breast footprint.
- Implant-associated anaplastic large cell lymphoma is rare but most commonly presents with a late seroma.
- Mastopexy and implant placement can be staged or performed together but have different risks depending on concurrence.
- Treatment of Poland's syndrome must adequately release fascial bands.

Questions

Breast Reduction

1. What is your approach to evaluating the patient with symptomatic macromastia (Fig. 13.1)?

Begin with a focused history and note the patient's current bra size and BMI, and a breast history, including how many times she has been pregnant, how many children she has, and how long she has breast fed—if at all. I note whether her breasts increased in size or decreased in size after breastfeeding. I ask about specific symptoms from the size of her breasts, such as back and shoulder pain, shoulder grooving from her bra straps, and intertrigo rashes, and how she has treated those conditions. I also ask about family history of breast or ovarian cancer, any breast masses or nipple discharge, if and when she had a mammogram.

2. When do you order a preoperative mammogram on a breast reduction patient?

The current (2015) American Cancer Society (ACS) screening recommendations are the option of a baseline mammogram at age 40 years and screening beginning at age 45 years for healthy women. The ACS does not recommend stopping screening based on chronological age, but does note that screening may be stopped if a patient has a life expectancy of 3 to 5 years, has severe functional limitations, or has comorbidities that significantly affect life expectancy. In those cases, a patient would likely not be a candidate for an elective breast reduction.

Alternative guidelines are the U.S. Preventative Service Task Force, an independent group that, under the auspices of the Department of Health and Human Services, used predictive modeling to aid in creating recommendations. Their recommendations are routine screening of average-risk women starting at age 50 years and continuing to age 74 years.

3. How do you examine a patient for a breast reduction?

First, evaluate the breasts, noting any asymmetry and the grade of ptosis she has. Grades of ptosis, as classified by Regnault, are as follows: grade I—the nipple-areolar complex (NAC) is at the inframammary fold (IMF); grade II—the NAC is below the

IMF; and grade III—the NAC is at the lowest portion of the breast. Pseudoptosis is when the NAC is in the appropriate position but the glandular tissue is below the IMF (**Table 13.1**).

I palpate for masses and check for nipple discharge, and take the following measurements: chest circumference in inches, bust circumference in inches, breast width in centimeters, sternal notch to nipple in centimeters, NAC diameter in centimeters, and nipple to IMF in centimeters (**Table 13.2**).

4. The patient wants to know whether she can breastfeed after the procedure. What do you tell her?

While there is no guarantee that one can breastfeed after a breast reduction, some studies have shown that equivalent percentages of women can breastfeed as those who have not had breast reduction, when the NAC is not attached as a free nipple graft. A free nipple graft would not allow breastfeeding.

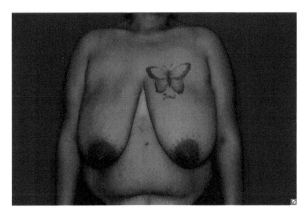

Fig. 13.1 A patient presents with complaints of large breasts.

Table 13.1 Classification of breast ptosis

Grade I breast ptosis	Nipple at the level of the inframammary fold (IMF)
Grade II breast ptosis	Nipple below the IMF
Grade III breast ptosis	Nipple at the lowest contour of the breast
Pseudoptosis	Glandular tissue below IMF

Table 13.2 Breast measurements

Breast measurement	Units	Utility
Chest and bust circumference	Inches	Can help assess whether patient is wearing correct bra size
Breast width	Centimeters	Determines horizontal breast footprint. Wide breasts are less likely to have narrowing after reduction, and may appear as less of a reduction
Sternal notch to nipple	Centimeters	A marker of ptosis as well as asymmetry
Nipple to inframammary fold	Centimeters	A marker of ptosis, asymmetry, and can be used to determine whether a free nipple graft is needed

5. What technique do you use for a breast reduction?

I use a vertical technique with a supero-medial pedicle. The technique is a combination of the skin resection pattern, and the pedicle.

RATIONALE: A breast reduction pattern has two components: the skin resection pattern and the pedicle design. Skin resection patterns can be combined with different pedicle designs. There are two classic skin patterns: the Wise pattern, or "anchor scar," and the vertical pattern (or "snowman"). The pedicle—the breast tissue that remains and through which the NAC receives its blood supply—can be based inferiorly, superiorly, medially, superomedially, laterally, or centrally. The inferior pedicle is very common, and many of the measurements to determine a free nipple graft are based on the inferior pedicle. A study by van Deventer demonstrated a robust blood supply to the NAC from the internal mammary artery.[1]

A posterosuperior pedicle is rarely used, but can be based off the anterior intercostal artery perforators.[2]

6. In which circumstances would you choose an inferior pedicle over a superior pedicle or superomedial pedicle?

Because the superior pedicle and supero-medial pedicles raise the IMF, I would use an inferior pedicle if the IMF needed to remain the same or be lowered.

7. Under what circumstances would you perform a free nipple graft?

The indication for a free nipple graft are very large, very ptotic breasts, and—in some cases—tobacco use. While previous recommendations were to consider a free nipple graft with a nipple–IMF distance of greater than 18 cm that does not take into account patient variation, and that measurement speaks to inferior, rather than medial or superomedial pedicles.

8. The NAC is so large that you cannot resect all of the areolar skin in your pattern. What do you do?

The NAC skin that cannot be resected is left to allow for wound closure. I would talk with the patient preoperatively about the area, and could plan for staged resection after healing.

9. You perform a breast reduction using a superomedial pedicle and a vertical skin resection. Intraoperatively, the NAC appears dusky. What do you do?

With intraoperative NAC duskiness, the viability can be assessed using fluorescein.

10. On postoperative day 1, the NACs appear slightly dusky. What do you do?

First, I loosen the sutures. If the NACs do not become more pink, I would consider using nitropaste. If these do not work, I would take her back to the operating room (OR) and convert to a free nipple graft. A free nipple graft can be successful if performed within 48 hours of the original operation.

11. What do you tell the patient about a free nipple graft?

I would counsel her that she will lose sensation, and that breastfeeding (if she is planning on having more children) is not possible. Some hypopigmentation is expected with a free nipple graft. A free nipple graft is likely to be successful even if the NAC was congested on the pedicle because the graft can survive by imbibition until inosculation occurs.

Breast Augmentation

1. Describe what you expect to see in a patient who presents for routine cosmetic breast augmentation.

The patient would likely have small breasts without signs of significant asymmetry.

2. What do you offer her?

I would offer implants.

3. How do you decide which implants to use?

Saline implants feel less natural than silicone, but do not require monitoring the way that silicone implants require monitoring.

Food and Drug Administration (FDA) recommendations are that patients with silicone implants undergo MRI 3 years after placement of the implants, and every 2 years after that.

There have been no studies that have shown an association of implants with rheumatologic disorders.

4. How do you decide whether to place them in the subglandular or submuscular position?

In patients with a very thin skin envelope, I would recommend submuscular placement. In patients with a thicker skin envelope, subglandular implants are acceptable. This is determined by performing a pinch test with calipers at the upper pole where the implant will be. If there is less than 2 cm of tissue, a submuscular technique should be used. If the pinch is greater than 4 cm, a subglandular technique can be used.[3] A modification of the subglandular approach is to place it under the fascia of the pectoralis muscle. This helps cover the edges of the implant, which can be palpable or visible in thin patients.

Assessing the five parameters of *coverage, implant volume, implant dimensions, IMF location*, and *incision location* as described in the "High Five Decision Support Process," published by Tebbetts and Adams,[4] will help in deciding whether to place the implant in the subglandular or submuscular position.

5. How do you decide the incision to use?

I prefer an inframammary incision, because it allows wide exposure, the incision is hidden underneath the curve of the breast, and there is less risk of contamination and sensory changes when compared with the periareolar and transaxillary approaches. In clothes, it is also covered. It is placed approximately 1 cm above the IMF and is at least 3 cm for a saline implant and at least 4.5 cm for a silicone implant.

6. Do you give antibiotics postoperatively?

There is no evidence to support giving antibiotics postoperatively for breast implant placement. There is currently only graded D evidence (level V) regarding continuation of antibiotic prophylaxis in expander implant reconstruction beyond the Surgical Care Improvement Project (SCIP) guidelines of 24 hours.[5]

7. The patient returns to clinic 7 weeks after the implant is placed, and her breast is hot and swollen. What do you do?

First, I would get a history and examine her, and find out if she has systemic evidence of infection, such as fevers, and I would establish a time line of symptoms course. I would perform a physical examination looking for fluid collections, and the extent of the erythema. If there is a fluid collection, I would take her to the OR.

If there is no fluid collection, and the time course has been short, I would give a trial of IV antibiotics.

8. Which antibiotics would you use?
The specific antibiotics that would be appropriate are dependent on the nomograms at my institution. We treat with vancomycin and Zosyn for broad-spectrum coverage. If there is significant improvement after 24 hours, we transition to oral antibiotics, and use ciprofloxacin or levofloxacin.

9. She does not improve after antibiotics. What do you do?
I would explore the pocket and remove the implant. I would also send cultures from the OR.

10. After the implant is removed, it is replaced several months later. She returns to your clinic several years later and reports that one breast appears fuller than the other. What do you do?
I would evaluate for a seroma. If there is a seroma, I would send her for ultrasound-guided biopsy of the fluid collection and send the fluid for cytology to rule out anaplastic large cell lymphoma (ALCL).

11. She is worried about ALCL. What do you tell her?
The overall risk of ALCL is low, and ALCL is 2% of non-Hodgkin's lymphomas. In a study in the Netherlands, there were a total of 11 cases of ALCL in the breast over a span of 17 years.[6] There does appear to be an increased risk with breast implants, but there is evidence that ALCL associated with breast implants behaves differently than other systemic forms, and may be more indolent.[7,8]

12. She returns complaining that her breast is painful and firm. What do you do?
I would exclude a capsular contracture. Capsular contractures are risks with all breast implants, but textured implants have a lower risk of capsular contracture.[9] They have, however, a higher risk of ALCL.

13. What are her risks for capsular contracture?
For subglandular placement with smooth implants, the relative risk is increased compared with both textured implants and subpectoral placement.[9,10]

Mastopexy

1. What technique do you use for a mastopexy?
The technique is determined by the characteristics of the skin envelope of the breast as well as the degree of ptosis. A small amount of ptosis with skin excess would be appropriate for a skin-only mastopexy.

2. The patient states that she would like implants with her mastopexy. What do you tell her?
Mastopexy is staged with implants. This allows the skin envelope to retract without placing considerable strain on it. It also allows patients to give me a better idea of what size they would like. It is possible to conflate ptosis with lack of volume, and many patients find that they are satisfied with the volume after the mastopexy.

3. After 3 months, she returns and one NAC is higher than the other. What do you do?
Three months is still too soon for revision. Even if there is an asymmetry, the scars will continue to mature and a revision will be in a dynamic, rather than, static field.

4. She comes back after another 3 months and it is still asymmetric. What do you do?
I would offer her a revision, and because it is easier to raise an NAC than lower one, I would raise the lower NAC to match the higher one.

5. Will she have to pay for the revision?
Yes. The policy on revision is disclosed in the preoperative consent and financial paperwork. Asymmetry is a possible

postoperative event, and revisions require payment.

Tuberous Breast Deformity

1. Describe the defect.
The patient has a tuberous breast deformity with asymmetry, and the defect on the affected side is graded (**Table 13.3**). The anatomy is characterized by a vertically constricted base, hypoplasia of the breast tissue in one or more quadrants, an elevated IMF, and herniation of the breast parenchyma into the areola.

The tuberous breast is characterized by herniation of breast tissue into the areola, while the tubular breast has a constricted base but no herniation.

The critical features in the assessment of the tuberous breast are the extent of the skin envelope deficiency, and the extent of soft-tissue deficiency. A skin envelope deficiency will require that the skin be expanded, and a parenchymal deficiency can be addressed by auto-augmentation, implant reconstruction, or a combination of the two.[11,12]

2. What is your initial step in management?
I would first assess her development and confirm that her growth has stopped, and assess for Poland's syndrome.

3. What is Poland's syndrome?
Poland's syndrome is a birth defect characterized by unilateral underdevelopment or agenesis of the chest wall, and can include agenesis of the sternal head pectoralis major muscle. It is also associated with syndactyly of the ipsilateral hand, and can be associated with shortened ribs.

4. Does the presence of Poland's syndrome change your management?
It does not change the management of the breast deformity, but it does impact the counseling given to the patient and the expected results of surgery.

5. What do you offer the patient?
If there is not an adequate skin envelope, tissue expansion is an option. In type II and III breasts, I would discuss with the patient whether she is happy with the size of her breasts. If there is adequate tissue, Ribeiro's technique combines a circumareolar incision with autoaugmentation using an inferior pedicle. The NAC is maintained on a superior pedicle, and an inferior flap is made by dividing the lower pole from the upper pole of the breast, making sure to disrupt the fascial ring. The inferior flap is then folded inferiorly to provide lower pole fullness. This technique can be modified; **Fig. 13.2** shows the sequence of an autoaugmentation. An implant can be placed either subpectorally or subglandularly.[12]

6. Where do you place the implant?
I would place the implant in the subpectoral position. While it is acceptable to

Table 13.3 Grading of tuberous breast deformity

Tuberous breast grade	Hypoplasia
I	Inferomedial quadrant
II	Inferomedial and inferolateral quadrants, adequate areolar skin
III	Inferomedial and inferolateral quadrants, adequate areolar skin
IV	All quadrants

Adapted from von Heimburg D, Exner K, Kruft S, Lemperle G. The tuberous breast deformity: classification and treatment. Br J Plast Surg 1996;49(6):339–345 and Grolleau JL, Lanfrey E, Lavigne B, Chavoin JP, Costagliola M. Breast base anomalies: treatment strategy for tuberous breasts, minor deformities, and asymmetry. Plast Reconstr Surg 1999;104(7):2040–2048

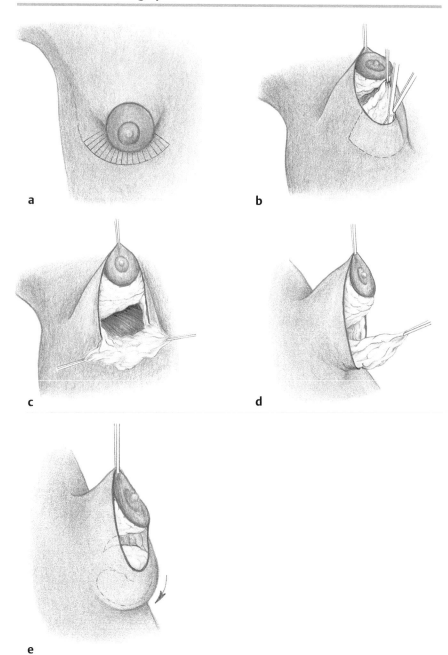

Fig. 13.2 Fullness can be provided in correction of tuberous breasts by repositioning native tissue. Implant techniques can be used with or without repositioning of breast parenchyma. (From Gabka CJ, Bohmert H. Plastic and Reconstructive Surgery of the Breast. 2nd edition. Stuttgart: George Thieme Verlag; 2009.)

place the implant in the subglandular position, this position can result in a persistent deformity, and can sometimes cause the appearance of two IMFs.

7. Do you use a saline or a silicone implant?

A saline implant has the advantage of some intraoperative adjustment of size. While a silicone implant may feel more natural, the lack of ability to make small adjustments to size on the table would decrease the ability to obtain good symmetry.

8. The patient has a persistent deformity. What most likely happened?

Most likely, it was inadequate release of the constricting fascial bands, and lack of release of the IMF and not enough radial scoring of the breast .

References

1. van Deventer PV. The blood supply to the nipple-areola complex of the human mammary gland. Aesthetic Plast Surg 2004;28(6):393–398
2. Mojallal A, Moutran M, Shipkov C, Saint-Cyr M, Rohrich RJ, Braye F. Breast reduction in gigantomastia using the posterosuperior pedicle: an alternative technique, based on preservation of the anterior intercostal artery perforators. Plast Reconstr Surg 2010;125(1):32–43
3. Heden P. Breast augmentation. In: Guyuron B, Eriksson E, Persing J, et al, eds. Plastic Surgery: Indications and Practice. London: Elsevier Saunders; 2008
4. Tebbetts JB, Adams WP. Five critical decisions in breast augmentation using five measurements in 5 minutes: the high five decision support process. Plast Reconstr Surg 2005;116(7):2005–2016
5. Alderman A, Gutowski K, Ahuja A, Gray D; Postmastectomy Expander Implant Breast Reconstruction Guideline Work Group. ASPS clinical practice guideline summary on breast reconstruction with expanders and implants. Plast Reconstr Surg 2014;134(4):648e–655e
6. de Jong D, Vasmel WLE, de Boer JP, et al. Anaplastic large-cell lymphoma in women with breast implants. JAMA 2008;300(17):2030–2035
7. Roden AC, Macon WR, Keeney GL, Myers JL, Feldman AL, Dogan A. Seroma-associated primary anaplastic large-cell lymphoma adjacent to breast implants: an indolent T-cell lymphoproliferative disorder. Mod Pathol 2008;21(4):455–463
8. Kim B, Roth C, Chung KC, et al. Anaplastic large cell lymphoma and breast implants: a systematic review. Plast Reconstr Surg 2011;127(6):2141–2150
9. Headon H, Kasem A, Mokbel K. Capsular contracture after breast augmentation: an update for clinical practice. Arch Plast Surg 2015;42(5):532–543
10. Wong CH, Samuel M, Tan B-K, Song C. Capsular contracture in subglandular breast augmentation with textured versus smooth breast implants: a systematic review. Plast Reconstr Surg 2006;118(5):1224–1236
11. von Heimburg D, Exner K, Kruft S, Lemperle G. The tuberous breast deformity: classification and treatment. Br J Plast Surg 1996;49(6):339–345
12. Grolleau JL, Lanfrey E, Lavigne B, Chavoin JP, Costagliola M. Breast base anomalies: treatment strategy for tuberous breasts, minor deformities, and asymmetry. Plast Reconstr Surg 1999;104(7):2040–2048

14 Back and Trunk Reconstruction

Abstract

This chapter will review back and trunk reconstruction for defects cause by trauma and tumor resection. The reader will be able to outline a management plan, draw incision for local flaps, and present alternative reconstructions in the case of wound recurrence.

Keywords: back reconstruction, myelomeningocele, sternal defect

Six Key Points

- Back defects can often be covered with local flaps.
- Sternal wounds can be covered with pectoralis flaps, rectus abdominis flaps, or omental flaps.
- Thoracic defects can be covered with latissimus flaps if the blood supply hasn't been interrupted.
- Infected mesh must be removed.
- Infected mesh does not need to be replaced if a capsule has formed.
- Free flap coverage is an option if blood supply is interrupted to regional flaps.

Questions

Case 1

A Plastic Surgery consult is placed for management of a myelomeningocele in a neonate (**Fig. 14.1**)

1. What do you see?

There is a large sacral wound in a neonate. Other things to note about its appearance are its posture, particularly its flexed position, and it has a difference in color between the upper half and the lower half of the body, similar to a harlequin baby.

2. Why is the color significant?

Neonates, and in particular neonates with myelomeningocele, have autonomic dysfunction that may lead to abnormalities in perfusion. This is particularly significant in a child with a myelomeningocele because an inferiorly based flap may have difficulty with perfusion.

3. Why is the posture significant?

The posture can signify what the long-term mobility may be. Some patients with myelomeningocele are ambulatory, while some are confined to a wheelchair. In a patient confined to a wheelchair, planning of the operation must balance coverage needs and preservation of functional muscle, including latissimus.

4. Neurosurgery is planning to take the child to the operating room. How do you plan coverage?

The first-line coverage that I would use is local flaps. It is important to know how neurosurgery is planning to cover the dura—with a primary repair or with a graft. If there is a graft, there must be vascularized tissue over the defect.

5. What flap do you use?

For this defect, bilateral rotational flaps.

6. Draw it.

The drawing can be seen in **Fig. 14.2**.

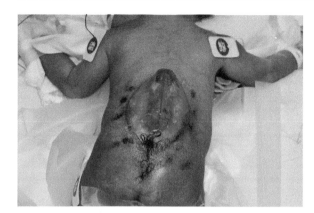

Fig. 14.1 A 1-day-old newborn referred for reconstruction.

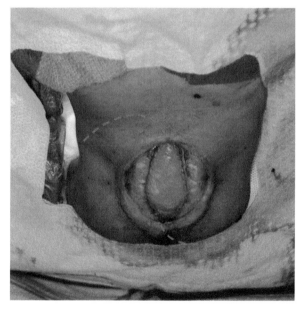

Fig. 14.2 Red dotted lines indicate planned incisions for coverage of a myelomeningocele defect.

7. Do you take fascia or latissimus muscle with the flaps?

Because the fascia and the muscle are so thin in a 1-day-old neonate, it is difficult to take fascia. The latissimus muscle is also very thin. In this case, it is best to preserve the latissimus both as a lifeboat in case the flap does not survive and as a functional muscle for mobility in a wheelchair. Paraspinous muscle can be turned over for coverage.

8. What are operative considerations with paraspinous muscle?

Paraspinous muscle is also an option for coverage, and in fact in a 15-year review accounted for 40% of dural coverage.[1] Elevation and rotation of the paraspinous musculature must be performed in consultation with neurosurgery, as in some cases the nerve roots can have anomalous courses and elevation of the paraspinous musculature must take that into account.

9. What are other options for designs of flap coverage?

Other designs include unilateral or bilateral rhomboid flaps, and other rotational flap designs such as a Yin-Yang design (**Fig. 14.3**).

10. How do you counsel the parents about postoperative complications?

Parents are informed of postoperative complications, which can include skin edge separation, flap separation, flap necrosis, cerebrospinal fluid (CSF) leak, pseudomeningocele, hematoma, seroma, and infection.

11. The nurse calls on postoperative day 2 and states that there is a small amount of clear sticky fluid coming out of the wound. What do you do?

The first step is to confirm that it is not CSF. After involving neurosurgery, if there is enough of a sample it can be sent for analysis for beta-2 transferrin,[2] although that test can take some time. If it is, the patient may be a candidate for a shunt.

12. It is not CSF fluid. What do you do?

It is then managed conservatively with local wound care and daily examinations to confirm it is not developing into a seroma.

13. The nurses call you and state there appears to be a wound separation on postoperative day 4. What do you do?

The first step is to evaluate the wound. If it is a small separation, additional nylon sutures can be placed at the bedside. If nylon sutures will not hold the tissue together, wet to dry dressing changes can be used or silver sulfadiazine can be used.

14. The nurses call and state that the tip of the left-sided flap looks dusky. What do you do?

After observing the extent of the duskiness and evaluating for surrounding cellulitis and fluid collections, it is most appropriate to treat conservatively.

15. The nurses are concerned that the dural repair is showing.

The dural repair, if vascularized, can be managed conservatively. Some authors describe placing skin grafts over the dural repair, although without infection or CSF leak, conservative management is appropriate at this time.

Case 2

A Plastic Surgery consult is placed for coverage of the defect shown in **Fig. 14.4**

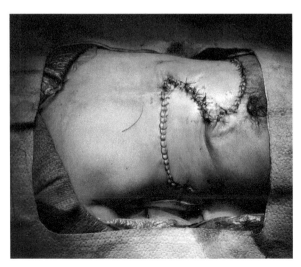

Fig. 14.3 Appearance after closure using "Yin-Yang" rotational flaps.

1. What is your perioperative management of sternal dehiscence?

Preoperatively, the patient should have a CT scan to evaluate for mediastinitis—the signs of which are sternal destruction, fluid, abscess pockets, and mediastinal widening. The patient should have laboratory studies including a complete blood count, blood cultures, and c-reactive protein.

2. How do you know a sternal infection has been adequately debrided?

There should not be visible necrotic tissue, and all tissues should appear healthy and be bleeding. The bone should be firm and the bone edges should have punctate bleeding. Cultures, both swabs of the deep pocket and bone biopsies, should be sent for culture, and the total wound size should be measured (**Fig. 14.5**).

3. The cardiothoracic surgeons have requested coverage. What do you do?

The first-line choice for coverage is bilateral pectoralis major advancement flaps.

4. The left internal mammary artery (IMA) has been harvested for cardiac bypass. Does that change your management?

No. While harvesting the IMA can affect a turnover flap based on the IMA, it will not affect an advancement flap based on the thoracoacromial artery.

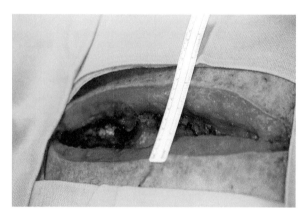

Fig. 14.4 Sternal wound. The top of the picture is cranial and the bottom of the picture is caudal.

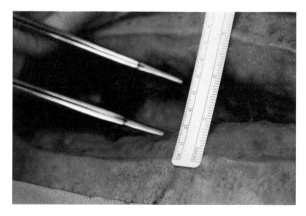

Fig. 14.5 Once a sternal wound is debrided to healthy tissue, and prewash and postwash cultures have been taken, the wound is measured.

5. Describe the procedure.

The suprafascial plane is identified and a skin and subcutaneous flap, which does not include the pectoralis fascia, is made for several centimeters. The pectoralis major muscle is identified at its medial aspect and the muscle in its entirety is elevated off of the chest wall. The thoracoacromial pedicle is identified at the superior aspect of the muscle and lies at the intersection of the midclavicular line (junction of middle and lateral thirds of clavicle and xiphoacromial axis). The muscle is released from its lateral attachments and advanced into the defect.

6. The muscle doesn't reach. What do you do?

If it is known before the dissection how much is needed, a rectus fascia extension can be taken inferiorly. The insertion of the pectoralis muscle can be released through a small counterincision in the axillary crease. If this is still not enough to cover the defect, then omentum can be harvested, or rectus abdominis muscle can be used for the lower part of the defect.

7. Five months later, the patient presents to the clinic with a draining sinus. What do you do?

While the presumptive diagnosis is underlying sternal infection, imaging can help identify abscesses and any bony destruction.

8. What imaging do you get?

A CT scan will show abscess pockets as well as some signs of osteomyelitis. A fistulogram may help identify if the sinus tract communicates with the bone.

9. The fistulogram does not show communication with bone. What do you do?

Even without communication with bone on fistulogram, the presumption is that the sinus tract is caused by bony infection. Thus, the treatment will be bony debridement.

10. You debride the bone and send cultures. What do you do?

The previous flaps are carefully raised to be replaced. If additional tissue is needed, an omentum or rectus abdominis can be used. If there is concern that the bone will need to be re-debrided, a negative pressure wound therapy can be placed.

Case 3

A thoracic surgeon requests coverage of the lateral chest wall, in which old scar and tumor is present.

1. What are you going to do?

In this case, free flap reconstruction is appropriate. A pedicled latissimus flap can be unavailable for two reasons: first, because the blood supply has been compromised through a previous incision and, second, because the muscle will be harvested with the resection. A pedicled rectus flap can be used for some coverage but may not cover the entirety of the defect, as the maximal dimensions of the muscle are 30 cm × 10 cm. An ALT flap can be used for coverage, and although the dimensions for primary closure are 25 cm × 8 cm, the donor site can be skin grafted if a larger area is needed.

2. The chest wall is reconstructed with methylmethacrylate mesh. Does this change the plan?

No. The mesh needs to be covered with vascularized tissue.

3. How do you monitor the flap post-op? What is your post-op protocol?

The flap is monitored with an internal Doppler and with hourly flap checks for the first day, and on post-op day 2 they are converted to every-2-hour flap checks.

4. The patient returns to the clinic 1 month after surgery, and is doing well. She wants to know if she can participate in full activity.

Yes, 1 month after surgery she can be released to full activity.

5. She returns to clinic 4 months after surgery and states a small area has opened up and is draining clear liquid. What do you do?

The first concern is that this is a draining sinus tract, signifying infection of the mesh. The first step is to evaluate the wound for signs of overt infection, such as cellulitis, purulent drainage, or fluid collections.

6. There are none. What do you do?

A fistulogram can be performed to see if there is communication with the mesh, but a negative study will not rule out an infection, so I would not order it routinely unless thoracic surgery needed it for planning. A draining sinus needs to be presumed to be associated with infected mesh.

Thoracic surgery needs to be asked if the infected mesh can be removed. If the mesh is removed, often a thick capsule has formed around the mesh by 4 months' time, such that no further bony reconstruction needs to be done. The ALT flap would be elevated such that the pedicle is not disturbed, and would be replaced in the same position after the mesh has been removed.

References

1. Lien SC, Maher CO, Garton HJL, Kasten SJ, Muraszko KM, Buchman SR. Local and regional flap closure in myelomeningocele repair: a 15-year review. Childs Nerv Syst 2010;26(8):1091–1095

2. Mantur M, Łukaszewicz-Zając M, Mroczko B, et al. Cerebrospinal fluid leakage: reliable diagnostic methods. Clin Chim Acta 2011;412(11–12): 837–840

15 Aesthetic Body and Trunk

Abstract

This chapter will review aesthetic surgery of the trunk and body, including abdominoplasty, liposuction, brachioplasty, and thighplasty. Readers will be able to identify physical examination findings that can be addressed with aesthetic surgery of the body and trunk, draw and describe operative incisions and techniques, formulate postoperative protocols, and manage complications.

Keywords: abdominoplasty, brachioplasty, thighplasty

Six Key Points

- Abdominoplasty is distinct from panniculectomy in that it includes rectus plication.
- Whether liposuction can be performed at an ambulatory facility is determined by the amount aspirated.
- Postoperative fluid shifts in liposuction must be monitored.
- Liposuction and brachioplasty or thighplasty can be staged.
- Care for the postliposuction, fluid-overloaded patient is supportive.
- Widened scars for brachioplasty and thighplasty are common, and are monitored and revised as needed.

Questions

Case 1

A patient presents the following in **Fig. 15.1**.

1. What do you do for this patient?

In a patient with infraumbilical lipodystrophy, an abdominoplasty will help with the abdominal contour by removing excess skin and fat, and correcting a rectus diastasis.

The evaluation begins with an assessment of the patient's history, including pregnancy history and any history of abdominal surgery. Social history, including tobacco use, is also assessed. A physical examination includes an assessment of rectus diastasis as well as any evidence of hernias.

Assuming the patient is a nonsmoker, otherwise healthy, is not obese, and has no evidence of hernias, an abdominoplasty can be offered as an outpatient procedure.

2. Describe the operative procedure.

The patient is marked in the standing position. The midline is marked from the xyphoid process to the pubic bone. Any asymmetries are noted to the patient. The inferior extent of the incision is marked, and the lateral aspect measured to ensure symmetry. The superior aspect of the incision is tentatively marked, and any areas of liposuction are marked.

The patient is placed supine on the operating room table, and prepped and draped. The inferior incision is made, and electrocautery is used to dissect through subcutaneous fat to rectus abdominis fascia. Scarpa's fascia is identified during the dissection. Once the rectus fascia is identified, the dissection proceeds cranially. Over the anterior superior iliac spine, the lateral femoral cutaneous nerve is identified and protected, or a layer of fat is left over the anterior superior iliac spine to protect it. Once the region of the umbilicus is reached, a knife is used to incise the skin around the umbilicus. Either electrocautery or Metzenbaum scissors are used to dissect around the stalk to the

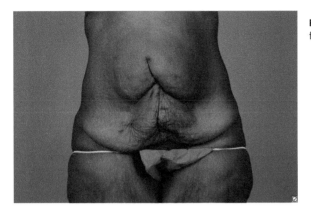

Fig. 15.1 A patient presents for abdominoplasty.

abdominal wall. Once the umbilicus has been isolated, the dissection proceeds superiorly in a triangle shape such that wide undermining is not performed laterally. The diastasis is corrected by imbricating the diastasis and sewing it closed with 0 polypropylene suture and then over-sewing it again. The abdominal flap is advanced, the excess skin is removed, and the incision is closed in layers after drain placement.

3. Postoperatively, she calls to report that her umbilicus appears dark. What do you do?

The umbilicus must be evaluated in person. "Duskiness" indicates venous congestion, and some degree can be expected. If it is dusky on examination, I would recommend conservative management with dressing changes.

4. She is doing dressing changes, and states that it has turned into a scab. What do you do?

The umbilicus can still be managed conservatively. If there is loss of some of the umbilicus, it can still be managed conservatively and will granulate.

RATIONALE: A 2006 study in the *Journal of Plastic, Reconstructive, and Aesthetic Surgery* reviewed complication in abdominoplasties[1] and noted that 18% of patients had early complications, and skin necrosis represented 1.5% in the early complications

category. Overall, early complication rates are 18 to 32%, although not all complications require revision.

Case 2

1. A patient wants liposuction of her abdomen. What do you do?

Liposuction is most appropriate for patients who have localized lipodystrophy and whose skin has good elasticity. In a patient with abdominal, thigh, or flank lipodystrophy, liposuction may be appropriate.

2. The patient states she has read about laser liposuction and would like that done. What do you tell her?

There are several different ways to perform liposuction. Suction-assisted lipectomy is traditional liposuction, which uses a cannula attached to a vacuum source. Ultrasound-assisted liposuction uses ultrasound, which first liquefies the fat and tissue, followed by traditional liposuction, and is useful for dense tissue, such as a gynecomastia correction. Laser-assisted liposuction uses varying wavelengths to help produce adipocyte lipolysis, and skin contraction, thought to be mediated by neocollagenesis. Currently 1,064-, 1,320-, and 980-nm diode laser-assistant liposuction machines are available.[2] Wither laser-assisted liposuction confers any benefit over other techniques has not been clearly established—some studies have failed to show any advantage other than reduction in pain and lipocrit levels.[3]

3. How do you counsel the patient about the risks?

There are several categories of risks of liposuction. First, there are intraoperative risks of bleeding, infection, lidocaine toxicity, and abdominal viscera perforation. In the immediate postoperative period, there are the risks of fluid shifts and fat embolism. Postoperatively, there are risks of contour irregularity and seroma.

4. Where do you perform the operation?

The operation can safely be performed in an outpatient setting; however, indications to perform surgery in an inpatient facility include large-volume liposuction and patient-specific factors such as obstructive sleep apnea.

Rationale: While there are no randomized controlled trials addressing this topic, there are currently restrictions at the state level regarding the circumstances under which liposuction can be safely performed at an outpatient facility. Some states restrict the amount of aspirate to 1,000 mL. The American Society of Plastic Surgeons (ASPS) consensus statement is that in the absence of more restrictive state guidelines, liposuction with aspirate greater than 5,000 mL should be performed in an acute-care hospital.

5. What technique to do you use for tumescence?

The tumescent technique, in which 3 mL of infiltrate is infused to 1 mL of aspirate, is appropriate for non–large volume liposuction. For large-volume liposuction, a super-wet technique in which 1 mL of infiltrate is infused for each milliliter of aspirate is appropriate to reduce the risk of fluid overload.

6. How do you do the procedure?

Under general anesthesia, the patient is given perioperative antibiotics and has deep vein thrombosis (DVT) prophylaxis with sequential compression devices placed.

7. In the postanesthesia care unit, the nurse calls you to tell you that the patient has a higher-than-usual blood pressure. What do you do?

The first step is to evaluate the patient at the bedside and confirm the vital signs. A higher-than-usual blood pressure can indicate pain, which would need to be assessed, and can also indicate fluid overload. Other signs of fluid overload are pulmonary symptoms such as a cough, dyspnea, and crackles on auscultation.

8. If the patient is fluid overloaded, what do you do?

Care is supportive. The patient would need to be admitted for observation, and a Foley catheter placed. Diuretics can be given as needed, although this can be controversial and potassium levels must be monitored during treatment.

9. The patient returns 2 months postoperatively and complains that there is contour irregularity. What do you do?

Contour irregularities are the most common complication of suction lipectomy. This can be prevented by the following: not using suction until the cannula has been inserted, cross-tunneling from separate sites, fanning, and using small-diameter cannulas near the surface. Immediately postoperatively, it is appropriate to continue to monitor it, as there can still be swelling. If it persists after 1 year, fat grafting can be performed to the irregularities.

Case 3

A patients presents the following in **Fig. 15.2**

1. What do you offer the patient?

A traditional brachioplasty can be offered to the patient and can reduce the circumference of the arms.

2. How do you decide which type of brachioplasty to perform?

The decision of which type of brachioplasty to perform is based on the presence of excess fat and the amount and location of skin laxity. In patients with excess fat but no skin laxity, liposuction may be appropriate. In patients with excess skin in the proximal third of the arm, a limited medial brachioplasty can be performed. If the excess skin extends to the chest wall, an extended brachioplasty is performed. If the excess skin includes the entire upper arm but does not extend to the chest wall, a traditional brachioplasty is performed.

RATIONALE: The algorithmic approach to brachioplasty takes into account fat as well as excess skin.

3. Where do you design your incisions?

The incisions can be designed in the bicipital groove.

4. Describe the procedure.

The patient is marked in the standing position and placed supine on the operating room table with the arms abducted. Antibiotic and DVT prophylaxis is instituted. The upper extremities, axillae, and shoulder are prepped into the field. After the patient is prepped and draped, local anesthetic is infiltrated into the incision sites. The superior incision is made and dissection is in the subcutaneous plane, deep to Scarpa's fascia but leaving 1 cm of fat on the muscle fascia. As the dissection proceeds distally, fat is left on

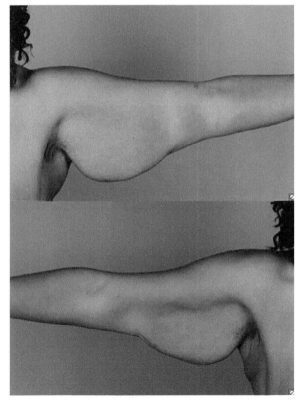

Fig. 15.2 A patient presents for a brachioplasty.

the muscle fascia to protect the medial antebrachial cutaneous nerve. Once the flaps have been created, the final resection is not performed until closure is confirmed. Closure is performed by anchoring the superficial fascial system with interrupted sutures. Drains are placed, and the skin is closed in layers.

5. What is your postoperative protocol?
Postoperatively, the drains are kept in place until the output is less than 30 mL/d. The arms are kept wrapped with an ACE (All Cotton Elastic) bandage.

6. Postoperatively, she complains of paresthesias of her left arm. What do you do?
The first step in evaluation is to determine whether there is injury to the medial antebrachial cutaneous nerve, which is subfascial in the bicipital groove in the proximal two-thirds of the arm, and pierces the deep brachial fascia approximately 14 cm proximal to the medial epicondyle. The nerve is most often adjacent to the basilica vein.

The dissection leaves approximately 1 cm of fat along the muscle fascia, to protect the nerve. To the extent that the nerve was identified and protected, it may be a neuropraxia and I would counsel her to monitor the area.

If the nerves were transected and a painful neuroma develops, a neuroma excision may be necessary. The neuroma can be identified by the presence of a Tinel sign over the injured nerve. The nerve is identified, and the end is buried in muscle.

Case 4

A patient presents the following in **Fig. 15.3.**

1. How do you assess the patient?
The first step is to identify the history, including whether there has been massive weight loss, whether the patient has a history of wound healing problems and diabetes mellitus, and whether the patient has a history of lower extremity swelling. In addition, the DVT risk is calculated. Lower extremity swelling can worsen after a thighplast.

2. What procedure do you offer?
In this patient, a staged thighplasty with liposuction first, to reduce the amount of subcutaneous tissue, followed by a formal thighplasty, can lead to the largest reduction in excess skin and fat. Liposuction and thighplasty can also be performed together.

3. Where do you design your incisions?
The incisions can be designed as vertical incisions. The APEX (anterior proximal extended) thighlift can be used in massive weight loss patients who have skin laxity in the proximal portion of the thigh. The incisions are designed in the inguinal crease and the infragluteal crease.[4]

4. Describe the procedure.
The patient is taken to the operating room and placed supine on the operating room table. DVT prophylaxis is initiated with sequential compression devices. The patient receives perioperative antibiotics and if liposuction is to be performed, it is performed. For the thighplasty, the anterior-most incision is made, and electrocautery is used in the subcutaneous plane. Once the flap has been raised, it is advanced, and the tissue is not resected until closure can be confirmed.

5. What is your postoperative protocol?
The postoperative protocol for thighplasty must take into account the risk of thigh swelling and DVT. The patient should wear leg wraps with ACE bandages or garments to help with swelling, and DVT prophylaxis

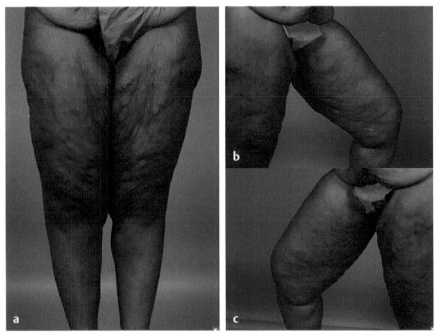

Fig. 15.3 A patient presents for a thighplasty. (**a**) Frontal and (**b,c**) medial views of the thighs are shown.

should be considered based on the Caprini score.

6. The patient returns 1 month later and complains of asymmetry. What do you do?

Most patients have some asymmetry pre-operatively, which is documented in the chart and in the preoperative photographs. There can also be asymmetric swelling. It is important to give the patient enough time for the swelling to decrease.

7. After 1 year, the patient still complains of asymmetry. What do you do?

One year is usually adequate time for the tissues to equilibrate. After 1 year, any asymmetry will likely last. Contour deformities are usually a result of technique, whereas asymmetry may be due to preoperative asymmetry. In both cases, revision surgery can be considered after 1 year.

References

1. Stewart KJ, Stewart DA, Coghlan B, Harrison DH, Jones BM, Waterhouse N. Complications of 278 consecutive abdominoplasties. J Plast Reconstr Aesthet Surg 2006;59(11):1152–1155
2. Goldman A, Gotkin RH. Laser-assisted liposuction. Clin Plast Surg 2009;36(2):241–253, vii, discussion 255–260
3. Prado A, Andrades P, Danilla S, et al. A prospective, randomized, double-blind, controlled clinical trial comparing laser-assisted lipoplasty with suction-assisted lipoplasty. Plast Reconstr Surg 2006;118:1032–1045
4. Shermak MA, Mallalieu J, Chang D. Does thighplasty for upper thigh laxity after massive weight loss require a vertical incision? Aesthet Surg J 2009;29(6):513–522

16 Pressure Ulcers

Abstract

This chapter will review pressure ulcers and the preoperative optimization of flap candidates in pressure ulcer reconstruction. Readers will be able to diagnose pressure ulcers and plan the preoperative optimization and surgical intervention of pressure ulcers, as well as formulate postoperative protocols.

Keywords: pressure ulcer, osteomyelitis, flap surgery

Six Key Points

- First-line treatment for pressure ulcers is conservative management with pressure offloading and nutritional optimization.
- Presence of sensation, ambulatory status, and level of spinal cord injury are considerations.
- Evaluation should include assessment for previous surgery.
- Presence of palpable bone is an indication of osteomyelitis.
- Ischial debridement may lead to other pressure ulcers.
- Recurrence rates are high; surgery does not treat underlying problem.

Questions

Case 1

A T11 paraplegic presents with a pressure ulcer (**Fig. 16.1**).

1. What do you do?

The first step is to identify the location, the anatomic location of the pressure ulcer (in this case sacral), assess for previous surgery, either from known history or from visible scars, and then stage the pressure ulcer. After the pressure ulcer is staged, it is important to ascertain the circumstances surrounding the development of the pressure ulcer, and the patient involvement in a turning or moving protocol. Initial conservative steps should be taken to pack the wound with wet to moist dressing changes, turn the patient or move every 2 hours, improve nutrition, and optimize the patient's overall medical condition with tobacco cessation, strict blood glucose control, weight loss, a bowel regimen, and spasm control.

2. What are the indications to use a negative pressure wound dressing?

Negative pressure wound therapy can have the advantages of reducing the total number of weekly dressing changes and stimulating the development of granulation tissue. Contraindications include malignancy, presence of eschar or fibrinous material, exposed blood vessels or viscera, or fistulas with unknown distal drainage.

3. The patient has soilage of the pressure ulcer despite a strict bowel regimen. What do you recommend?

If there is persistent soilage despite a bowel regimen, the pressure ulcer will not heal. A diverting colostomy is indicated in those instances.

4. There is exposed bone. What do you do?

Exposed bone, or the ability to probe to bone, indicates the presence of osteomyelitis. The wound can still be treated

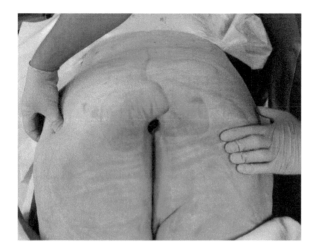

Fig. 16.1 Sacral pressure ulcer. Note that one must observe the patient and photograph carefully, as imprints from clothing and sheets can have the appearance of scars. (This image is provided courtesy of James Gatherwright, MD.)

Table 16.1 Options for pressure ulcer flap coverage

Location of pressure ulcer	Option 1	Option 2
Sacral	Superior gluteal artery flap	Transverse back flap
Ischial	Ambulatory: gluteal fasciocutaneous	
	Paraplegic below T12: TFL	
	Paraplegic above T12: Posterior thigh V-Y flap	
Trochanteric	Vastus lateralis	TFL

conservatively until the patient is optimized for surgery. Bone biopsies can be performed to guide antibiotic therapy.

RATIONALE: The "probe-to-bone" test has been validated for diagnosing chronic osteomyelitis in the diabetic foot.[1]

5. Would you resect the osteomyletic bone?
The amount of debridement that should be performed on bone is dependent on the location. The Trochanter can be debrided and some limited debridement of the sacrum can be performed. Limited bony debridement can be performed on the ischium. If a complete ischiectomy is performed, it will increase the obliquity during sitting, and will increase the risk of a pressure ulcer on the contralateral side. If bilateral ischiectomies are performed, then risks of perineal ulceration and pressure ulcer increase.

6. What flap do you use?
V-Y advancement flaps and rotational flaps can be used for sacral pressure ulcers (**Table 16.1**). Gluteal perforator flaps and V-Y advancement flaps can be used, and some of the medial skin can be de-epithelialized (**Fig. 16.2**). The ambulatory status of the patient is critical in deciding whether or not to use muscle.

Case 2

The patient pictured has a recurrent pressure ulcer (**Fig. 16.3**).

1. What do you do?
The first step, as in all pressure ulcers, is to identify the reason for the recurrence, and correctable factors. Once nutrition is optimized, and compliance with positioning is documented, surgery is considered if the

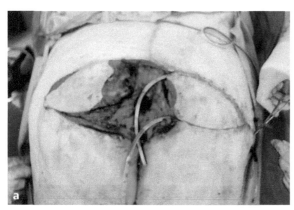

Fig. 16.2 Gluteal perforator V-Y advancement flap. Note how the skin can be (**a**) de-epithelialized and (**b**) inset. (These images are provided courtesy of James Gatherwright, MD.)

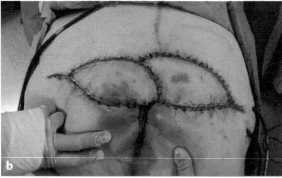

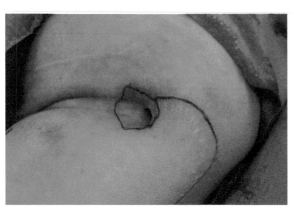

Fig. 16.3 Pressure ulcer recurrence. (This image is provided courtesy of James Gatherwright, MD.)

pressure ulcer remains inert despite optimization of nutrition and positioning.

The patient must demonstrate healing capacity, must not smoke, and should have a bowel regimen as well as control of urine. Any spasticity should be controlled.

2. What flap do you use?

If a prior rotational or advancement flap has been used, the first choice is to readvance the flap.

3. Draw it.

The flap is drawn as in **Fig. 16.4**.

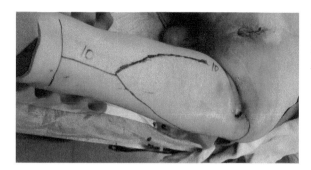

Fig. 16.4 Design of a flap for the pressure ulcer. (This image is provided courtesy of James Gatherwright, MD.)

4. What is your po.erative protocol?

Postoperatively, the patient spends 3 weeks on a low air loss bed, and the operative site is pressure free. Antibiotics are tailored to intraoperative bone biopsies and cultures. Drains are kept until the output is less that 30 mm/d, and care is taken that the patient is not lying on the drains, to avoid pressure from the drain tubing. The incision is dressed with bacitracin and gauze dressings.

After 3 weeks,[2] a sitting protocol is initiated in which the patient sits for 30 minutes and the flap is checked, and the sitting time increases in 30-minute increments.

References

1. Lam K, van Asten SA, Nguyen T, La Fontaine J, Lavery LA. Diagnostic accuracy of probe to bone to detect osteomyelitis in the diabetic foot: a systematic review. Clin Infect Dis 2016;63(7):944–948

2. Tchanque-Fossuo CN, Kuzon WM Jr. An evidence-based approach to pressure sores. Plast Reconstr Surg 2011;127(2):932–939

17 Traumatic Hand Injury

Abstract

Because specific trauma may vary, the chapter will provide an *approach* to the diagnosis and management of hand trauma using specific case examples, so that readers will feel confident addressing hand trauma that they may not have seen before.

Keywords: hand trauma, hand therapy

Six Key Points

- Assessment of hand injuries includes a systematic assessment and catalogue of injured structures.
- Identifying the injury/deformity is critical.
- Early institution of hand therapy protocols is necessary for hand injuries.
- The majority of postoperative hand-specific complications can be diagnosed by physical examination; imaging can be used as an adjunct.
- Intraoperative complications include loss of vascularity, and vasospasm should be treated with papaverine or lidocaine.
- Unrecognized injuries can lead to secondary deformities, such as a swan neck deformity after flexor digitorum superficialis rupture.

Questions

Case 1

A patient resents the injury in **Fig. 17.1**.

1. Describe what you see.

A laceration between the A1 pulley at the palm and the insertion of the flexor digitorum superficialis on the middle phalanx, with loss of active flexion of the distal interphalangeal joint (IPJ) and proximal IPJ, is most consistent with a Zone 2 flexor tendon laceration, of both the flexor digitorum profundus and flexor digitorum superficialis tendon.

2. What do you do?

Assuming that this is an isolated trauma and the patient has no other contraindications for surgical intervention, the ideal window to take the patient to the OR is within 72 hours. The patient should be consented for a primary tendon repair but be prepared for the possibility of a two-stage repair.

3. Describe your operative steps and explain how you repair the tendon.

The operation is performed under general anesthesia or an axillary block, and a padded pneumatic tourniquet is placed on the arm. The original laceration is identified, and Bruner zigzag incisions are designed such that the points of the incisions are on the radial or ulnar aspect of the finger at the flexion creases.

The neurovascular bundles are identified and retracted radially and ulnarly, and the tendon sheath is identified. The distal and the proximal stumps are identified.

4. You can't see the proximal stump. What do you do?

It is possible that the stump has retracted, depending on how flexed the finger was during the injury. The palm can be milked and this sometimes delivers the tendon.

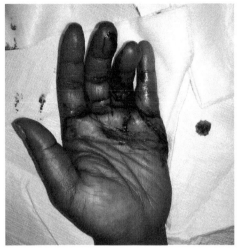

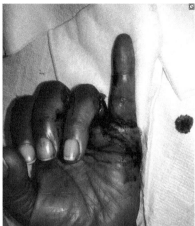

Fig. 17.1 Posture of hand after laceration (**a**) Resting posture and (**b**) an attempted fist formation.

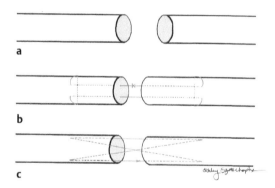

Fig. 17.2 Schematic of two-strand and four-strand core suture repairs for tendons. (**a**) The cut tendon edges. (**b**) The two-strand modified Kessler repair. (**c**) The four-strand cruciate repair. (Reproduced with permission of Ashley Szuter-Uncapher, Clinical Photographer.)

If this does not work, a small incision can be made at the level of the A1 pulley and a small catheter such as a pediatric number 8 feeding tube can be fed through the sheath, attached to the tendons, to deliver the tendon. This technique is described by Sourmelis and McGrouther.[1]

5. You find the proximal stump this way. How do you repair the tendon?

The tendon should be repaired with a four-strand core repair. Studies of sutures show that core suture strength is a function of three variables: type of suture, caliber of suture, and number of strands in the repair. A two-strand repair such as Kessler or modified Kessler is less strong than a four-strand repair such as a cruciate repair (**Fig. 17.2**), and an eight-strand repair is stronger than a four-strand repair.[2]

Ultimately, however, the bulk of the suture interferes with gliding. A four-strand repair, assuming that there is enough bulk of the tendon, is appropriate. Knots can be placed outside of the repair site.[3]

No more than 3 mm of gapping should be present, because it decreases strength of repair and increases the chance of rupture.

An epitendinous repair using a 6–0 Prolene will also increase strength.

6. What is your postoperative rehabilitation protocol?

The patient sees a hand therapist within 5 days after surgery, and the postoperative splint is changed for a dorsal-blocking splint with the wrist in neutral, metacarpophalangeal joints (MCPJ) in 70 degrees of flexion, and IPJs in up to 10 degrees of flexion. An early active protocol is initiated in which the patient performs place-and-hold exercises for 3 minutes in the splint, followed by passive flexion and active extension in the splint.

At 3 weeks, the splint can be removed for exercises, but remains in place otherwise. After 6 to 8 weeks, the splint can be removed in a controlled fashion.

An alternative program is the Duran passive motion protocol, in which all exercises are performed in the splint.

7. After 3 months, the patient is not moving his finger that much. What do you do?

The clinical question is whether the patient is not moving because of scar or rupture. An MRI may help elucidate the cause. If it is not clear from the MRI, the patient is consented for an exploration and a possible tenolysis versus a staged tendon reconstruction.

8. Describe a staged tendon reconstruction.

A staged tendon reconstruction is performed if the tendons can't be repaired primarily in the initial operation, for example, if there isn't enough skin coverage or if there is too much of a gap. Once there is stable soft-tissue coverage, a Hunter rod is sutured distally and is brought proximally to the level of the carpal tunnel. It can either be left free or sutured to proximal tendon.

The Hunter rod is left in place for 3 months, during which time a capsule forms around the rod.

After 3 months, a tendon graft is placed.

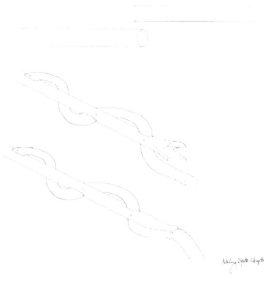

Fig. 17.3 Pulvertaft weave. A Pulvertaft weave is used to provide mechanical strength to a tendon graft or transfer. (Reproduced with permission of Ashley Szuter-Uncapher, Clinical Photographer.)

9. The patient does not have a palmaris longus. What do you use as a tendon graft?

A plantaris tendon, which can be harvested through an incision just anterior to the medial margin of the Achilles tendon and found between the gastrocnemius and the soleus, can be used. If the plantaris is not an option, the toe extensors or flexors can be used.

The tendon graft must be sutures using a Pulvertaft weave (**Fig. 17.3**).

Case 2

A 27-year old male flals while skiing and presents an injury to the thumb.

1. What is the diagnosis?

The mechanism of injury—a fall while using ski poles—and the laxity of the ulnar aspect of the thumb at the MCP joint are consistent with the diagnosis of an ulnar collateral ligament tear.

2. What do you do first?

After obtaining a full history of the injury including the time course, a full physical examination is performed.

The physical examination begins with inspection and palpation of the injured thumb. One expects to see tenderness and ecchymosis along the ulnar border of the thumb in an ulnar collateral ligament tear. It also includes an evaluation of the contralateral thumb and the ligamentous laxity. Laxity greater than 30 degrees at the ulnar collateral ligament is suggestive of an ulnar collateral ligament tear.

3. Is simply stressing the thumb enough to determine that the laxity is 30 degrees?

The volar plate contributes some stability, so the thumb should also be examined in approximately 40 degrees of flexion. Partial tears may have some degree of laxity, but complete tears will not have restriction on stress.

4. After examination, there is a bulge you did not feel before, near the injury. What happened?

This is most likely a Stener lesion, in which the adductor aponeurosis becomes interposed between the ligament and its insertion. Forceful manipulation can create a Stener lesion, and it can also occur after the injury itself.

5. What do you offer the patient?

In the case of a partial rupture, a trial of splinting with a thumb spica splint that immobilizes the MCP joint, for at least 4 weeks, can be attempted. A complete rupture will require operative repair.

6. How do you approach the operation?

After informed consent is obtained, and under tourniquet control, a lazy S incision is designed over the ulnar aspect for the thumb MCP joint, extending from the metacarpal to the proximal phalanx. Branches of the superficial radial nerve are identified and protected, and the proximal aspect of the adductor aponeurosis is dissected, and the Stener lesion, if present, is identified and placed back into its anatomic position. An incision is made in the adductor aponeurosis ulnar to the extensor pollicis longus. The ligament itself can be repaired with interrupted figure of eight sutures. The bony fragment can be captured with a Keith needle, which is passed through metaphyseal bone, and tied over a radial button.

7. A Keith needle is not available. What is another option for the bone?

Depending on the size of the fragment, a mini-fragment screw can be used, or a Kirschner wire.

8. What is your postoperative protocol?

The patient is placed in thumb spica cast for 4 weeks, and then begins hand therapy for range of motion. Outside of hand therapy, the patient remains in a thumb spica splint for 2 weeks. The repair is protected from stress, such as heavy lifting, for a total of 3 months.

9. The repair gets loose 6 months after the repair. What do you do?

Options for repair after rupture include reoperation and reinforcing the repair, or using a palmaris longus graft to reinforce or reconstruct the ulnar collateral ligament.

Case 3

A patient presents an injury to the thumb after a fall.

1. What is the diagnosis of the injury shown in Fig. 17.4?

An articular fracture of the base of the first (thumb) metacarpal, or Bennett's fracture.

2. What do you do?

Because the injury is a fracture subluxation, the fracture fragment remains in its anatomic position by the anterior oblique

ligament, while the metacarpal is dislocated by the action of the abductor pollicis longus, which subluxes the metacarpal proximally, radially, and dorsally.

A small fracture fragment (< 20% of the joint surface) can be treated with Kirschner's wire fixation of the metacarpotrapezial joint. Larger fragments are approaches through an open approach, and a Wagner incision that exposes the joint extends along the glabrous skin border of the thumb from the thumb metacarpal distally to the flexor carpi radialis proximally.

The fracture is exposed through incision of the metacarpal periosteum and exposure of the joint capsule.

The fracture fragment is reduced and a 2.0-mm lag screw is placed across the fracture fragments.

3. A lag screw is not available. What do you do?

If a lag screw is not available, semirigid fixation with two Kirschner's wires can be

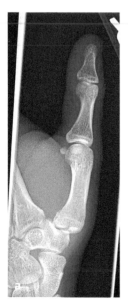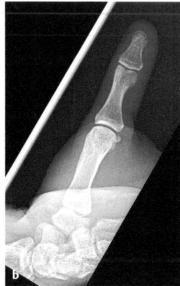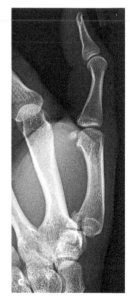

Fig. 17.4 Example of a Bennett's fracture. Note that the fracture is not seen well on all views. (These images are provided courtesy of Teresa Chapman, MD.)

used across the fracture fragments, with a transarticular Kirschner wire to help keep reduction of the entire complex.

4. What is the postoperative protocol?

The patient is maintained in a thumb spica cast for 1 month postoperatively, followed by hand therapy. Kirschner's wires are removed after 4 to 6 weeks, with radiograph confirmation of the reduction.

5. The patient returns 2 months later and reports persistent pain. What do you do?

The concern is a nonunion or malunion. Radiographs should be obtained to evaluate for a malunion. If there is a malunion, an osteotomy can be performed to re-create the fracture, and re-reduce it using the above protocols.

6. The patient returns with a persistent malunion and persistent pain. What do you do?

If a patient has failed attempts at correction, a carpometacarpal arthrodesis can be performed as a salvage procedure.

References

1. Sourmelis SG, McGrouther DA. Retrieval of the retracted flexor tendon. J Hand Surg [Br] 1987;12(1):109–111
2. Osei DA, Stepan JG, Calfee RP, et al. The effect of suture caliber and number of core suture strands on zone II flexor tendon repair: a study in human cadavers. J Hand Surg Am 2014;39(2):262–268
3. Norris SR, Ellis FD, Chen MI, Seiler JG III. Flexor tendon suture methods: a quantitative analysis of suture material within the repair site. Orthopedics 1999;22(4):413–416

18 Elective Hand Surgery

Abstract

This chapter will review common hand conditions for which elective surgery can provide treatment. Readers will be able to explain the management of each, and select appropriate postoperative hand therapy protocols.

Keywords: hand surgery, Dupuytren's contracture, first web space contracture

Six Key Points

- Elective hand surgery involves making a correct diagnosis and identifying all involved structures.
- Release of contractures may require soft-tissue coverage—know several options for coverage of the hand.
- Release of contractures requires night splinting to prevent recurrence.
- Postoperative assessment should include evaluation for inadvertent injury to critical structures.
- Postoperative protocols often include hand therapy.
- Indications for operative intervention always include a functional deficit.

Questions

Case 1

A patient presents the following in **Fig. 18.1**.

1. What do you see?
The photograph shows a flexion deformity of the finger with a visible cord. This is most consistent with Dupuytren's disease.

2. What do you do?
A history is taken that elicits concurrent pathology and factors associated with Dupuytren's, which include diabetes mellitus, alcoholism, smoking, and AIDS. In addition, factors associated with Dupuytren's diathesis are a family history of the disease, bilateral disease, multiple anatomic foci (such as plantar and penile lesions), and age younger than 50 years.

3. What are your indications to intervene?
Indications for intervention are a metacarpophalangeal joint contracture of greater than 30 degrees or a proximal interphalangeal joint (PIPJ) contracture of greater than 20 degrees, or a positive Hueston's tabletop test, in which the patient cannot put his hand flat on the table. Difficulty with activities of daily living often coincide with contractures of this degree.

4. What do you do?
With a palpable cord, collagenase injection can be administered. This is performed in the clinic, and the patient is consented for the procedure. The solution is injected into the cord, and the patient's hand is bandaged, and the patient is instructed his hand will swell and become bruised. The patient returns 1 to 3 days later for rupture.

5. After rupture, the patient has an appearance of the finger as in Fig. 18.2. What do you do?
Skin tears are common after cord release. One first checks for sensation if no digital

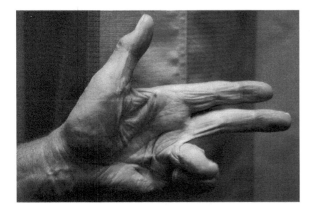

Fig. 18.1 Hand deformity. What is the diagnosis?

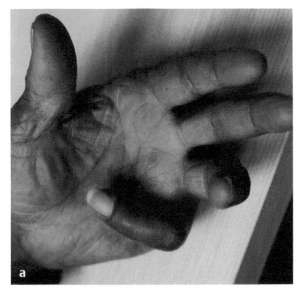

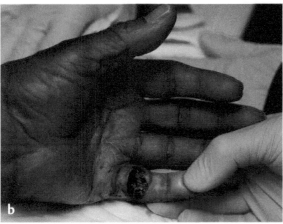

Fig. 18.2 Appearance of a finger (**a**) before (**b**) and after Dupuytren's release with collagenase.

block has been performed, to excluded nerve injury, and then independently checks flexor digitorum profundus and flexor digitorum superficialis function. An unidentified flexor digitorum superficialis injury can lead to a late swan neck deformity.

If no critical structures are injured, one treats the skin tear conservatively.

6. The patient doesn't want injections. What do you do?

Surgery is an alternative. The patient is consented for a palmar fasciectomy, and the risks of the procedure, including damage to the nerves and loss of blood supply to the finger, are discussed with the patient. Under tourniquet control, either Bruner incisions are made in the finger or the palm, over the cords, or straight-line incisions can be made with plans for Z-plasty. The dissection is made proximally with tenotomy scissors, and the cord and neurovascular bundles are identified. A transverse incision is made in the cord, and an approximately 1 cm segment is removed.

7. There is inadequate skin to cover the incisions. What do you do?

The wound can be left open, as with the McCash technique.[1] Alternatively, the area can be covered with a skin graft.

8. The cord to the PIPJ is released intraoperatively, and once the tourniquet is let down the finger appears white. What do you do?

The concern is vasospasm. The finger is first placed back into flexion. If that doesn't work, papaverine or lidocaine can be placed on the vessel.

9. The patient returns 2 days later and reports numbness in the finger. What do you do?

The clinical concern in this case is distinguishing between a neuropraxia from

stretching the nerve and a transected nerve. A physical examination is performed in which the radial and ulnar digital nerves are examined separated, and 2-point discrimination is assessed as well as sensation to pinprick, and Tinel's sign is checked along the course of the nerve.

A difference between the radial and ulnar digital nerves, dense paresthesias (particularly to pinprick), or Tinel's sign at the site of cord release are all suggestive of a nerve injury, and the patient is taken back to the OR for an exploration and possible release.

Case 2

A patient comes to clinic with an old burn scar of the first web space.

1. What is your diagnosis?

A first web space contracture can be diagnosed by history, physical examination, and appearance. In addition to skin contracture, adductor contractures can be present as well, and the basilar joint capsule can also be affected.

2. What do you offer the patient?

A "jumping man" flap is an option for first web space contractures, and is a five-flap modification of double-opposing Z-plasties.

3. Draw it.

The design is shown in **Fig. 18.3**.

4. What is your postoperative protocol?

The patient should be splinted with the thumb in abduction for 2 weeks, and then should wear a splint at night to prevent recontracture.

5. The patient returns 6 months later and has a recurrent contracture. What do you do?

Re-exploration to release all involved structures is the next step. If there is a significant soft-tissue defect, a reversed forearm

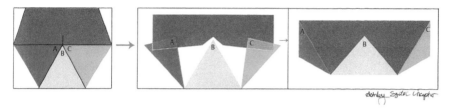

Fig. 18.3 Jumping man flap. (Reproduced with permission from Ashley Szuter-Uncapher, Clinical Photographer.)

flap is the procedure of choice. A posterior interosseous artery flap is a good choice for resurfacing. If that fails or is not an option, a radial forearm flap—assuming a patent palmar arch—is a good choice.

6. You perform a radial forearm flap, and 3 weeks after surgery the patient has exposed flexor carpi radialis. What do you do?
If the paratenon was left intact, the exposed tendon can be managed conservatively with dressing changes and the area should granulate. If there was no paratenon, the area can be bridged with a bilayer matrix of collagen–glycosaminoglycan biodegradable matrix.

Reference

1. McCash CR. The open palm technique in Dupuytren's contracture. Br J Plast Surg 1964;17:271–280

19 Lower Extremity Reconstruction

Abstract

This chapter will review the principles of lower extremity reconstruction after trauma. It will review preoperative assessment of blood flow and zone of injury, as well as reconstructive options. The readers will be able to analyze a given lower extremity injury and determine an appropriate operative intervention, and integrate the free flap failure algorithm in the management of postoperative complications.

Keywords: lower extremity reconstruction, zone of injury

Six Key Points

- Determine the etiology of the wound.
- Always assess the zone of injury.
- Determine baseline function and neurovascular status prior to reconstruction.
- Vascular integrity is key to lower extremity reconstruction.
- Post-operative rehabilitation protocols are key to a successful outcome
- Realistic expectations must be set for outcomes.

Questions

Case 1

A patient presents with an open leg wound after a motor vehicle crash. There is visible soft tissue loss.

1. What do you do?
The injury is at least Gustilo 3b injury, which can be identified by the size of the defect (> 1 cm) and periosteal stripping, which leaves the bone exposed. If there is associated arterial injury, the classification is a 3c injury. This classification is useful because type III injuries require flap coverage of bone (**Table 19.1**).

2. What do you do?
Assuming the patient is otherwise stable and orthopaedic surgery has adequately fixed the bone, preparations should be made for coverage. This begins with a full lower extremity examination, including motor and sensory function, and palpation of pulses.

Imaging is then ordered. An angiogram is ordered.

3. The angiogram is shown in Fig. 19.1. Describe what is in the angiogram.
The first vessel to come off of the popliteal artery is the anterior tibial artery, which appears the most lateral. The popliteal continues as the tibioperoneal trunk, and the next vessel, which appears medial to the anterior tibial artery, is the peroneal artery. The vessel then continues as the posterior tibial artery.

4. If only the posterior tibial vessel is open, what do you do?
In that case, the case is more complex, but an end-to-side anastomosis can be performed.

Table 19.1 Gustilo's and Anderson's classification of open tibial fractures

Gustilo type	Description
I	Wound < 1cm, no deep contamination
II	10 cm > wound > 1 cm without extensive soft-tissue damage
IIIA	Wound > 10 cm with soft-tissue coverage of bone
IIIB	Wound > 1 cm with exposed bone and periosteal stripping
IIIC	IIIB with arterial injury

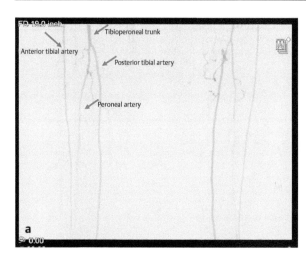

Fig. 19.1 Lower extremity angiogram. (**a**) Note how the peroneal artery becomes more diminutive as it travels distally. The red arrow in (**b**) points to an arterial blockage. It is important when evaluating angiograms to look not only at the runoff, but also for vessel caliber and any vascular pathology.

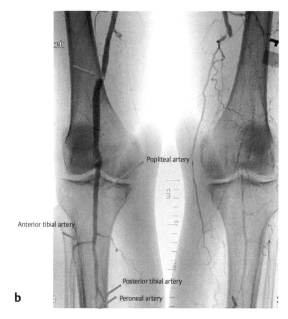

5. The end-to-side doesn't work. Are there any other options?

A staging of arteriovenous (AV) fistula to the proximal stump of an occluded vessel is an option.[1,2]

A staging of AV fistula is performed by anastomosing a vein graft, such as the saphenous vein, to a recipient artery and vein. The distal end is sutured to the artery and the proximal end to the vein, which creates a high-flow and low-resistance circuit. The procedure can be performed in one or two stages, and allows bridging of a defect.

6. The flap fails after 2 days, and salvage attempts are unsuccessful. What do you do?

The first step is to determine why it failed. The most likely reason that it failed in a trauma, assuming external causes of compression or kinking were excluded and the anastomosis was technically sound, was that the anastomosis was performed in the zone of injury.

7. What do you do?

Another flap can be performed, and a vein graft can be used to get out of the zone of injury.

8. Which vein do you use for a vein graft?

The saphenous vein is the most commonly used vein graft. Though some reports suggest an increased risk of failure with vein grafts, others demonstrate no increased risk.[3] The vein graft should be placed outside of the zone of injury, which can be determined by the presence of bleeding from side branches.

9. There is a bony defect. Does that change your management?

For limb salvage, wound control must be achieved first with stable soft-tissue coverage—in this case, a free flap. Once the wound is covered with vascularized tissue, bone grafting can be performed. Similarly, if tendon or nerve grafts are needed, they are performed after soft-tissue coverage is achieved.

Case 2

A patient presents a tibia wound.

1. What do you expect to see?

The proximal third of the tibia has an exposed wound, with an open area. Imaging should be reviewed, and shows callus and tibial periosteal elevation.

2. What is your management?

Initial management assumes the presence of osteomyelitis, and would involve an Infectious Disease consult for peripherally inserted central catheters (PICC) and IV antibiotics. If there is no malunion or nonunion, there may be no need for orthopaedic surgery involvement, but it is worthwhile to have orthopaedic surgery input regarding whether further orthopaedic surgery intervention is warranted.

3. Would you debride the wound?

Yes. One debrides starting with healthy tissue, using curettes and rongeurs, until there is healthy bone identified by a "crunch" and punctate bleeding.

4. You debride to healthy bone and it cracks. What do you do?

Ideally, orthopedic surgery would be called to place in external fixation and an antibiotic spacer, until there is soft-tissue healing.

5. How many weeks of antibiotics is required for osteomyelitis?

Six weeks of antibiotics is the standard for osteomyelitis.

6. How do you get soft tissue coverage?

For the proximal third of the leg, use a gastrocnemius flap (**Table 19.2**).

Table 19.2 Coverage options for the leg based on defect location

Defect location	Coverage	Pedicle
Proximal third of leg	Gastrocnemius	Medial sural artery and vein
Middle third of leg	Soleus	Popliteal, posterior tibial, and peroneal pedicles proximally and peroneal to distal lateral belly and posterior tibial to distal medial belly. The proximal vasculature supplies all but distal 4 cm of muscle.[4]
Distal third	Free flap Latissimus dorsi Rectus abdominis Gracilis Anterolateral thigh	Thoracodorsal artery Inferior epigastric artery Medial femoral circumflex artery—gracilis br. Lateral femoral circumflex—descending br.

7. You do a gastrocnemius flap and it doesn't quite reach. What do you do?
You can divide the origin.

8. It still doesn't reach. What do you do?
In that case, the option is a free flap.

9. Which free flap do you use?
A rectus abdominis has a long pedicle, and depending on the anatomy and the amount of dissection, 5 to 7 cm can be obtained for the pedicle. The artery itself has a diameter of 2 to 4 mm.

References

1. Lin CH, Mardini S, Lin YT, Yeh JT, Wei FC, Chen HC. Sixty-five clinical cases of free tissue transfer using long arteriovenous fistulas or vein grafts. J Trauma 2004;56(5):1107–1117

2. Cavadas PC. Arteriovenous vascular loops in free flap reconstruction of the extremities. Plast Reconstr Surg 2008;121(2):514–520

3. Classen DA. The indications and reliability of vein graft use in free flap transfer. Can J Plast Surg 2004;12(1):27–29

4. Raveendran SS, Kumaragama KG. Arterial supply of the soleus muscle: anatomical study of fifty lower limbs. Clin Anat 2003;16(3):248–252

20 Lower Extremity Wounds

Abstract

This chapter will review the management of chronic lower extremity wounds, including diabetic foot ulcers and chronic venous stasis ulcers. The reader will be able to identify the appropriate preoperative optimization and barriers to effective treatment of these wounds, and propose surgical management, as well as manage postoperative complications.

Keywords: lower extremity wounds, venous stasis ulcers

Six Key Points

- Wounds should be debrided and vasculature assessed.
- Chronic osteomyelitis may best be treated with a partial calcanectomy.
- One-half to two-thirds of the calcaneus can be removed surgically.
- Coverage can include local flaps with a partial calcanectomy or free flaps.
- Imaging should include plain films and MRI.
- Patients require orthotics.

Questions

1. What do you do with an open calcaneal wound (Fig. 20.1)?

Initially, the wound should be debrided. After that, a temporary dressing can be placed until the wound declares itself and full workup is completed.

2. What do you do next?

The vasculature should be assessed. If the patient is not renally impaired, and does not take metformin, an angiogram is appropriate. If no radiologic imaging can be done, then one should Doppler out the vessel. Noninvasive vascular studies should be performed, which can determine whether revascularization with vascular surgery should be performed first, or if the healing capacity is insufficient for salvage.

3. What next?

Once osteomyelitis has been treated, with either antibiotics or a partial calcanectomy, the wound should be covered.

4. How do you determine if a partial calcanectomy is an option?

Plain films will determine the amount of bony involvement, and MRI can be used as an adjunct to determine how much bone is involved. One-half to two-thirds of the calcaneus can be removed, but patients may require lifetime orthotics (**Fig. 20.2**).

5. How do you perform the partial calcanectomy?

Posterior or hockey stick incisions are used, and the skin flaps are dissected keeping their full thickness. Serpentine incisions can be used (the "hurricane" incision) if the surgeon wishes to avoid scarring of the posterior leg.[1] The Achilles tendon may be detached, and is preserved for reattachment later. The calcaneus is removed in a posterior-proximal/plantar distal with an oscillating saw or an osteotome. The remaining calcaneus is assessed for bleeding, and fluoroscopic appearance of sufficient bone. The Achilles tendon is reattached, with an anchor or with sutures.

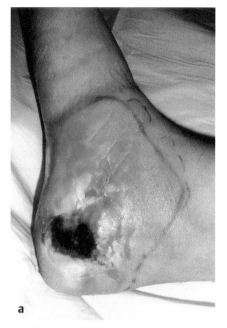
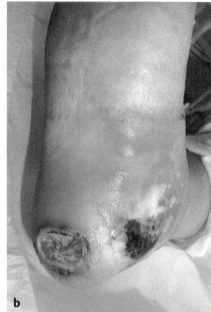

Fig. 20.1 A patient presents with a foot wound.

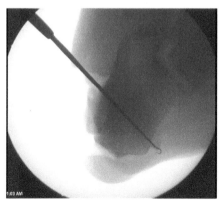
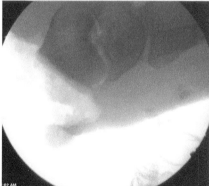

Fig. 20.2 Level at which a calcanectomy is performed.

6. The wound recurs after the partial calcanectomy. What do you do?

If there is no osteomyelitis, or the osteomyelitis has been treated, then a free flap can be considered if the vasculature is intact. The majority of successful free flap reconstructions are performed in trauma patients,[2] but can be considered in a patient with diabetes mellitus if the blood glucose is well controlled.

If the wound persists despite salvage attempts, the last option is an amputation.

References

1. Fisher TK, Armstrong DG. Partial calcanectomy in high-risk patients with diabetes: use and utility of a "hurricane" incisional approach. Eplasty 2010;10:e17

2. Kang MJ, Chung CH, Chang YJ, Kim KH. Reconstruction of the lower extremity using free flaps. Arch Plast Surg 2013;40(5):575–583

21 Cleft Lip and Palate

Abstract

This chapter will review unilateral and bilateral cleft lip, and cleft palate, with an emphasis on surgical markings. The reader will be able to categorize the defect and identify appropriate preoperative workup, and propose surgical plans and postoperative protocols. The reader will also be able to address postoperative events including dehiscence, fistulas, and velopharyngeal dysfunction.

Keywords: cleft lip, cleft palate, cleft lip and pala

Six Key Points

- The most important initial assessment is the airway.
- Cleft repair occurs along a standardized timeline.
- It is critical to understand and be able to draw cleft markings.
- The protuberant premaxilla should be controlled.
- Small lip dehiscences can be repaired primarily, while larger ones are left and revised after a year.
- Operative intervention for velopharyngeal dysfunction depends on the pattern of posterior and lateral wall movement.

Questions

1. What is your initial assessment of a child with cleft lip and/or palate?

Prenatal ultrasound detects over 90% of cleft lips. Many centers now have multidisciplinary cleft team evaluation of all infants with cleft lip with or without cleft palate, and presurgical assessment of an infant with cleft lip with or without cleft palate is threefold: airway, associated anomalies, and feeding and nutrition.

The most important initial assessment is of the airway—either at birth, or in the context of an airway history if the patient is being seen in clinic. If the airway is unstable, it needs to be stabilized with positioning, nasopharyngeal tubes, intubation, tongue–lip adhesion, or tracheotomy.

If the airway is stable, the infant should be evaluated for other anomalies, specifically cardiac and renal anomalies.

Finally, the infant needs a nutritional assessment. Some infants with cleft lip have difficulty latching onto a breast, although a nursing mother can often help create a seal over the cleft lip. Infants with cleft palate will not be able to create an oronasal seal, and will require a special nipple to obtain adequate nutrition. A pigeon nipple has a firm surface to abut the cleft, and a flexible surface for the tongue. The nipple is fitted with a one-way valve, which allows the infant to control and obtain fluid. Failure to thrive is a risk in children with clefts, and should be monitored.

2. What do you tell the parents?

The parents should be informed of the possible associated anomalies and feeding strategies, as well as the timing of repair.

3. What is the timing of surgery?

With cleft lip, if there is an alveolar cleft with a deformity of the alveolar arch, a lip adhesion with maxillary orthopaedics is performed at 6 weeks of age, followed by a definitive repair at 6 months. A single-stage palatoplasty is performed at 10 to 18 months. For cleft lip and palate, timing of surgery is around 10 weeks for the lip, and 10 to 18 months for the palate (**Fig. 21.1**, **Table 21.1**).

4. The family wants to wait until after the child is 18 months of age to repair the palate. What do you tell them?

The reason that cleft palate repair is performed before 18 months of age is because if the child cannot properly pronounce words, both speech and language acquisition will become disordered.

5. How do you control the premaxilla in bilateral cleft lip?

A protuberant premaxilla will need to be controlled. One can use preoperative orthodontics with passive presurgical molding or active molding, or bilateral lip adhesion. Passive molding is performed with nasoalveolar molding, which aligns the premaxilla with alveolar segments in bilateral clefts and aligns the alveolar segments in

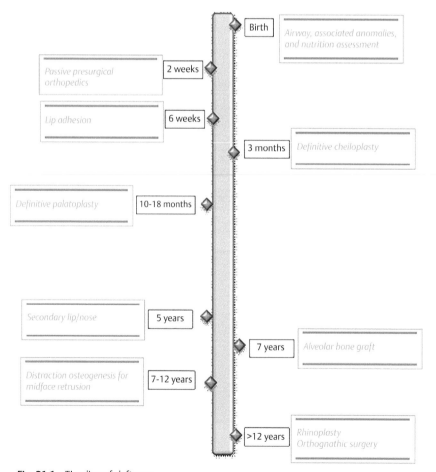

Fig. 21.1 Timeline of cleft care.

Table 21.1   Diagnosis, procedure associated with the diagnosis, and timing of the intervention.

Diagnosis	Procedure	Timing
Cleft lip and/or palate	Airway, associated anomalies, nutrition assessment	Birth
Alveolar cleft	Lip adhesion	6 wk
Cleft lip	Definitive cheiloplasty	6 mo
Cleft palate	Definitive cleft repair	10–18 mo

unilateral clefts. In addition, nasoalveolar molding uses nasal stents to mold the columella and nasal cartilage.

A Latham appliance is a device that is surgically inserted with pins, and is used to align the alveolus to make surgical repair easier. It is used for approximately 6 to 8 weeks.

6. When and how do you do a bilateral lip adhesion?

A bilateral lip adhesion can be performed at approximately 6 weeks of age. Bilateral lip adhesion is performed by raising 4 × 2 mm flaps bilaterally and suturing them together.

7. What is a maneuver you can use if the lip adhesion is tight?

You can put gentle pressure with your thumb on the segment to help reduce it. The risk with this maneuver is an infracture.

8. Draw the repair of a unilateral cleft lip.

The drawing can be made in the following steps (**Fig. 21.2**):

- **Step 1.** Mark the bilateral commissures, Cupid's bow peak on the noncleft side at the vermillion cutaneous border and its mirror image, along with its match on the lateral lip element. The base of the nostrils on the medial and lateral edge, the subnasale, and the midpoint of the Cupid's bow are also marked.
- **Step 2.** Once the landmarks have been marked, draw the rotation flap on the medial lip element. This is drawn from the mirror image of Cupid's bow peak arching toward the midpoint of the columella, and then making a sharp downward turn at the midpoint of the columella.

- **Step 3.** The advancement flap is on the lateral lip element by drawing a line from Cupid's bow peak match, along the cleft, and turning at the nasal sill.
- **Step 4.** The columellar flap is then made from Cupid's bow peak on the medial cleft element to the lateral columella.
- **Step 5.** The mucosal incisions are marked as extensions of the rotation and advancement flaps.

9. Draw the repair of a bilateral cleft lip.

The drawing is as in **Fig. 21.3**.

10. Draw the repair of a cleft palate.

The drawing is as in **Fig. 21.4**.

11. How do you manage the nose?

The degree of nasal deformity is assessed preoperatively. The length of the columella on each side is assessed, as the columella may be shorter on the cleft side. The cleft-side dome is flattened, with an obtuse angle, and the medial crus is shorter. The alar base is posterior and inferior. It is important to note that the alar cartilage is not simply malpositioned; it is also more atrophic.

The nose is exposed through the dissection. The alar base incision is extended to the inferior turbinates, and the alar cartilage is released from its lining and muscular attachments. The dissection continues to the noncleft side, and once the cartilage is free, the alar cartilage is shaped by placing polypropylene suture on Keith needles and Dacron pledgets through the dome to act as a handle. As this is lifted and the dome is shaped, a base stitch is placed through the orbicularis muscle, and an alar base suture is placed.[1]

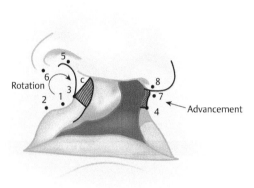

Fig. 21.2   Repair design of unilateral cleft lip. The steps are described in detail in the text. (From Woo AS. Plastic Surgery Case Review: Oral Board Study Guide. New York, NY: Thieme Medical Publishers; 2014.)

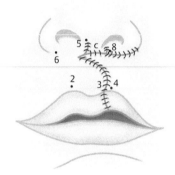

12. What is your postoperative protocol for a cleft palate repair?

After surgery, the patient is admitted to the hospital with Q3 hour flap checks. Bottle feeding is allowed immediately. Perioperative antibiotics are discontinued within 24 hours. Arm restraints are not necessary.

RATIONALE: A trial demonstrated that arm splints, though often used, are unnecessary after surgery.[2]

13. The lip dehisces. What do you do?

The first step in a lip dehiscence is to determine the cause. Common causes of lip dehiscences in cleft repair are a postoperative injury to the lip, tension on the repair from widely spaced cleft, or lack of a layered closure. If the area is small and the dehiscence can be repaired primarily without tension, it can be repaired soon after injury. If it cannot be repaired without

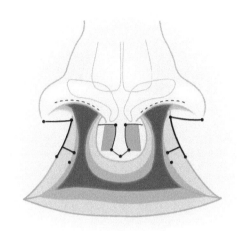

Fig. 21.3 Repair design of bilateral cleft lip. (From Woo AS. Plastic Surgery Case Review: Oral Board Study Guide. New York, NY: Thieme Medical Publishers; 2014.)

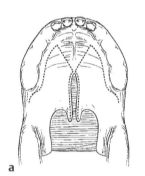
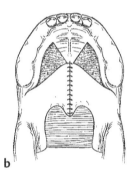

Fig. 21.4 Repair design of a cleft palate. (From Park SS. Facial Plastic Surgery: The Essential Guide. New York, NY: Thieme Medical Publishers; 2005.)

a b

tension, it is allowed to heal for at least 6 months to a year, and a secondary revision is performed after that.

14. The patient develops a palatal fistula. What do you do?

A palatal fistula can be a significant problem. There are several ways to address it. The first step is to readvance the flaps.

15. That fails - what do you do next?

Buccal musculomucosal flaps can be used for repair, and there are modifications such as folding the flap that can help simplify it.[3] A tongue flap can also be used.[4] Finally,

acellular dermal matrix can be used to repair a palatal fistula.[5]

16. How do you assess speech after cleft palate repair?

Speech is assessed at age 5 to 7 years. Diagnostic modalities include direct perceptual evaluation, nasendoscopy, and fluoroscopic evaluation.

17. The patient has been diagnosed with velopharyngeal dysfunction. What do you do?

The intervention for velopharyngeal dysfunction depends on the motion of the pharyngeal walls. There are three surgical interventions for velopharyngeal dysfunction: the Furlow palatoplasty, a pharyngeal flap, and a sphincter pharyngoplasty.

A Furlow palatoplasty is used to lengthen the palate, where there is good movement of the walls but the palate is too short (**Fig. 21.5**).

A pharyngeal flap elevates pharyngeal tissue and places it posteriorly (**Fig. 21.6**). This technique is useful when there is good lateral wall motion, because it adds bulk posteriorly and allows the lateral walls to reach the buttressed tissue.

A sphincter pharyngoplasty is appropriate for patients with poor posterior and lateral wall movement (**Fig. 21.7**).

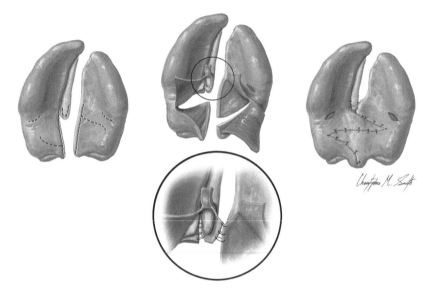

Fig. 21.5 Design of Furlow's palatoplasty, or double-opposing Z-plasty. (From Losee JE, Kirschner RE. Comprehensive Cleft Care. 2nd edition. New York, NY: Thieme Medical Publishers; 2016.)

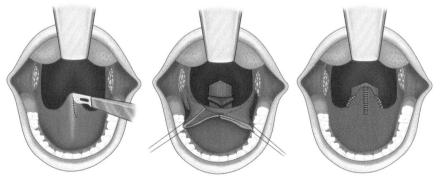

Fig. 21.6 Velopharyngeal flap incision design and inset for velopharyngeal dysfunction. (Adapted from Setabutr D, Senders C. Surgical Management of velopharyngeal dysfunction. Oper Tech Otolaryngol 2015;26(1):33–38.)

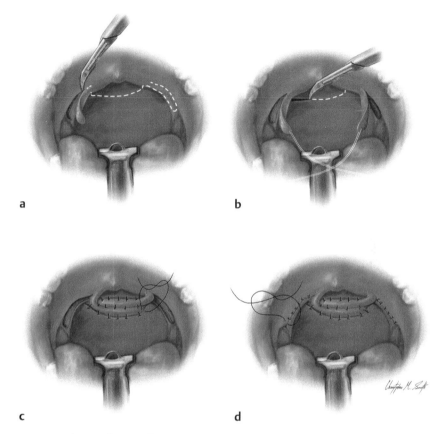

Fig. 21.7 Sphincter pharyngoplasty incision design and inset for velopharyngeal dysfunction. (From Losee JE, Kirschner RE. Comprehensive Cleft Care. 2nd edition. New York, NY: Thieme Medical Publishers; 2016.)

References

1. Marchac AC, Michienzi JW, Salyer KE. Unilateral cleft lip repair. Chapter 38. In: Chung KC, Disa JJ, Gosain AK, Kinneym BM, Rubin JP, eds. Plastic Surgery: Indications and Practice. Philadelphia, PA: Saunders Elsevier; 2009

2. Jigjinni V, Kangesu T, Sommerlad BC. Do babies require arm splints after cleft palate repair? Br J Plast Surg 1993;46(8):681–685

3. Kobayashi S, Fukawa T, Hirakawa T, Maegawa J. The folded buccal musculomucosal flap for large palatal fistulae in cleft palate. Plast Reconstr Surg Glob Open 2014;2(2):e112

4. Charan Babu HS, Bhagvandas Rai A, Nair MA, Meenakshi. Single layer closure of palatal fistula using anteriorly based dorsal tongue flap. J Maxillofac Oral Surg 2009;8(2):199–200

5. Losee JE, Smith DM. Acellular dermal matrix in palatoplasty. Aesthet Surg J 2011;31(7, Suppl):108S–115S

22 Craniosynostosis Syndromes

Abstract

This chapter will review craniofacial syndromes, with an emphasis on diagnosis and development of surgical management plans. The reader will be able to identify coexistent pathology and create timelines of surgical management and interventions.

Keywords: craniosynostosis, plagiocephaly, surgical management

Six Key Points

- Children with craniofacial syndromes should be assessed for anomalies in other organ systems.
- Assessment of the airway is the most important initial step.
- Neurocognitive outcomes are always a consideration.
- Timing of surgery is informed by osseous growth.
- In airway compromise unresponsive to intervention, tracheostomy should be considered.
- Distraction osteogenesis of the jaw should take into account tooth development.

Questions

Case 1

1. What would you see in a photograph of a child with unilateral coronal craniosynostosis?
The orbit in unilateral coronal craniosynostosis is differently shaped from one side to the other, with the eyebrow superiorly displaced on the affected side, and the nose and chin deviated toward the affected side. The shape of the orbit is called a harlequin deformity. The ear is anterior and superior on the affected side.

2. How do you distinguish this from nonsynostotic plagiocephaly?
In nonsynostotic plagiocephaly, or deformational plagiocephaly, the appearance of the skull is a parallelogram (**Fig. 22.1**).

3. The mother calls and reports that the patient is tilting his head. What do you do?
Children with unicoronal craniosynostosis can have head tilting because they have strabismus of the ipsilateral superior oblique muscle. I would have the patient see ophthalmology.

4. What operation do you offer the patient?
For unicoronal craniosynostosis, a fronto-orbital advancement is recommended at the age 4 months.

5. Why 4 months? Why not when the child is older?
There is some controversy in the literature. Some of the works by Marchac et al demonstrate that earlier intervention is prone to relapse, but later intervention (after 1 year of age) is associated with worse neuropsychological outcomes.[1]

6. The parents ask about cognitive outcomes. What do you tell them?
There are several issues relating to neuropsychological outcomes. The first is how craniosynostosis compares to the nonsynostotic

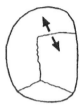

Synostotic anterior plagiocephaly

Synostotic posterior plagiocephaly

Deformational posterior plagiocephaly

Fig. 22.1 Comparison of unicoronal synostosis, lambdoid synostosis, and deformational plagiocephaly. (Adapted from Janis JE.Essentials of Plastic Surgery. 2nd ed. New York, NY: Thieme Medical Publishers; 2014)

population. The second is how outcomes correlate to the timing of surgery, and the third is how the choice of operation influences the outcomes.

When compared to normative samples, nonsyndromic craniosynostosis is associated with cognitive, speech, and behavioral abnormalities.[2] This is not predictive for any single child, but it does point to a need for longitudinal assessments and early intervention.

Early intervention is associated with better neuropsychological outcomes when compared to later intervention (after 1 year of age).[3]

Some researchers have documented better neuropsychological outcomes from cranial vault remodeling compared to strip craniectomy for sagittal synostosis.[4]

7. What do you counsel the patients about complications?

Complications of cranial vault remodeling include both aesthetic and neurosurgical complications. Aesthetic complications include poor cosmetic outcomes or relapse of the deformity, which has been shown to occur more with left-sided unicoronal craniosynostosis than with right-sided unicoronal craniosynostosis.[5] Neurosurgical outcomes include dural leaks, sagittal sinus injury that may lead to venous infarction, increased intracranial pressure, subdural hemorrhage, and increased intracranial pressure.

It is also important to counsel parents about the potential for blood transfusions in craniosynostosis repair. Craniosynostosis is associated with significant blood loss because of bleeding from venae emissariae.

Case 2

1. What would you see in a photograph of an infant with Pierre Robin Sequince?

A newborn infant with mandibular deficiency. Mandibular deficiency can be further characterized as hypognathia, retrognathia, or micrognathia.

2. What do you do?

There are two issues to address immediately. The first is to determine airway patency, and determine if any immediate intervention needs to be taken for the airway. The second is to determine any associated abnormalities and syndromic diagnoses that would inform prognosis and potentially require other interventions, such as cardiac interventions (**Table 22.1**).

3. The child has no evidence of other syndromes. What is your diagnosis?

A thorough physical examination would demonstrate findings consistent with syndromes. Physical examination assesses the airway, and the maxillomandibular discrepancy is measured by using a wooden stick and placing it at the apex of the mandibular alveolar ridge, and measuring the distance to the apex of the maxillary alveolar ridge.[6]

Table 22.1 Syndromes associated with micrognathia and morphological features

Syndromes associated with micrognathia	Other morphological features
Pierre Robin sequence	Cleft palate, high arched palate with or without a cleft, and glossoptosis
Treacher Collins	Colobomas, zygomatic hypoplasia, downward slanting eyes
Hemifacial microsomia	Hypoplasia of soft and hard tissue of face, can be unilateral or bilateral, auricular deformities
DiGeorge	Cardiac anomalies, palatal defects, velopharyngeal dysfunction
Cri du chat	Microcephaly, hypertelorism, epicanthal folds, low-set ears, cardiac anomalies

With mandibular deficiency, glossoptosis, and a high-arched palate, the most likely diagnosis is Pierre Robin sequence.

4. There is concern about airway patency. What do you do?

The initial step is to perform a thorough physical examination, and to obtain multidisciplinary data from providers in plastic surgery, pediatric otolaryngology, pediatric sleep medicine, pulmonology, anesthesia, and speech therapy. Pulse oximetry is used to check for desaturations, operationally defined as 5% or more of the time spent with SaO_2 less than 90% or any SaO_2 less than 80%.

If the infant has no desaturations, a formal sleep study is undertaken, and if the infant has no sleep disturbances and no desaturations with feedings, then observation is performed. If there are any sleep disturbances or desaturations with feedings, the infant undergoes nasoendoscopy and bronchoscopy.

If there is infraglottic or glottis obstruction, the child will need a tracheostomy. If, however, there is supraglottic or tongue-based obstruction, the first maneuver is positioning in the prone or lateral position. If the infant still has desaturations, a tongue–lip adhesion may be used.

5. Describe a tongue–lip adhesion.

A tongue–lip adhesion is performed by making an incision in the labial sulcus, exposing the orbicularis oris. A curvilinear incision is then placed on the undersurface of the tongue, exposing the muscles of the tongue. The labial and tongue mucosal flaps are then sutured to one another. The tongue is then suspended by placing sutures at the base of the tongue, and placed through the anterior portion of the tongue and suspended underneath the chin. A button or a silicone tube can be used at the base of the tongue to prevent the suture from pulling through.

6. The parents are worried that a button might become dislodged and the infant will choke. What is an alternative?

Some authors have described alternatives to using a button by creating a woven suture at the base of the tongue.[7]

7. What is your postoperative protocol after a tongue–lip adhesion?

The infant is monitored with pulse oximetry in the Intensive Care Unit (ICU). Assuming that there are no further desaturations, once the child is discharged home they are evaluated in clinic in 1-month intervals, and at each visit the maxillomandibular discrepancy is remeasured, and the tongue is assessed for movement. When the discrepancy is less than 3 mm, and the tongue has some muscular maturity, the tongue–lip adhesion is reversed. This may take up to 7 months of development.

Table 22.2 Timeline for distraction osteogenesis

Phase	Timing	Events during phase
Osteotomy/corticotomy phase	Time of surgery	
Latency phase	5–7 d	No turning, soft callus forms 3–7 d
Distraction phase	1–3 wk	Turn 0.25 mm every 6 h or 0.5 mm twice a day for 1 mm/d
Consolidation phase	3–4 mo	Turning arms removed but distractor in place
Remodeling phase	After removal of distractor	Functional loading

Note: The timeline can vary with age and the latency phase in infants is shorter than in children older than 2 years.

8. A tongue–lip adhesion is unsuccessful in stopping the desaturations. What do you do?

If a tongue–lip adhesion has been unsuccessful, the next step is distraction osteogenesis. Distraction osteogenesis is performed in the operating room and requires osteotomies of the mandible and placement of hardware with an external turning mechanism.

9. How do you counsel the patient's parents about the risks?

There is a risk that the distraction will interfere with tooth growth, and there could be risks of hardware infection, poor bone formation, and need for tracheostomy.

10. Five weeks out from the original surgery, after removal of the turning arms, they state that an area of the anterior mandible looks red. What do you do?

One evaluates the child for hardware exposure. If there is some hardware exposure, one treats with antibiotics. It is important to distinguish a true infection from erythema from irritation, and a true cellulitis will be bright red (**Table 22.2**).

If it is a true infection, one assesses how long the consolidation phase has been. If the consolidation phase has been at least 3 months, one can remove the hardware. If it has not been 3 months, one should consider consulting infectious disease to treat with suppressive antibiotics until the consolidation phase has ended.

11. The hardware needs to be removed early. What is the risk?

The risk is that the patient will have relapse.

12. The hardware is removed, and the patient has subsequent airway compromise. What do you do?

The patient would then need a tracheostomy.

References

1. Marchac D, Renier D, Broumand S. Timing of treatment for craniosynostosis and facio-craniosynostosis: a 20-year experience. Br J Plast Surg 1994;47(4):211–222

2. Becker DB, Petersen JD, Kane AA, Cradock MM, Pilgram TK, Marsh JL. Speech, cognitive, and behavioral outcomes in nonsyndromic craniosynostosis. Plast Reconstr Surg 2005;116(2):400–407

3. Arnaud E, Meneses P, Lajeunie E, Thorne JA, Marchac D, Renier D. Postoperative mental and morphological outcome for nonsyndromic brachycephaly. Plast Reconstr Surg 2002;110(1):6–12, discussion 13

4. Hashim PW, Patel A, Yang JF, et al. The effects of whole-vault cranioplasty versus strip craniectomy on long-term neuropsychological outcomes in sagittal craniosynostosis. Plast Reconstr Surg 2014;134(3):491–501

5. Becker DB, Fundakowski CE, Govier DP, Deleon VB, Marsh JL, Kane AA. Long-term osseous morphologic outcome of surgically treated unilateral coronal craniosynostosis. Plast Reconstr Surg 2006;117(3):929–935

6. Schaefer RB, Stadler JA III, Gosain AK. To distract or not to distract: an algorithm for airway management in isolated Pierre Robin sequence. Plast Reconstr Surg 2004;113(4):1113–1125

7. Mann RJ, Neaman, KC, Hill, BH, Bajnrauh, R, Martin, MD. A novel technique for performing a tongue-lip adhesion: the tongue suspension technique. Cleft Palate Craniofac J 2012;49(1):27–31

Appendix A: Practice Photos

The following are select photographs of defects. Copy and draw your repair designs. Suggested reconstructions for 1-8 appear in **Appendix B**. Try to solve the rest on your own.

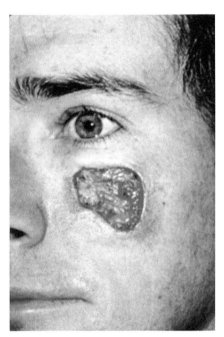

A1 from Cheney M, Hadlock T, ed. Facial Surgery: Plastic and Reconstructive. 1st Edition. Thieme; 2014.

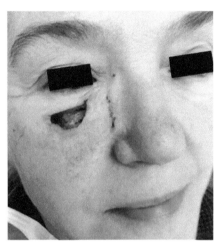

A2 from Quatrano N, Stevenson M, Sclafani A, et al. V-Y Advancement Flap for Defects of the Lid-Cheek Junction. Facial Plastic Surgery. 2017; 33(03):329-333.

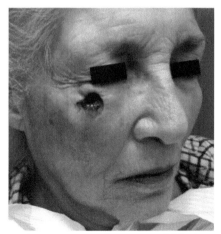

A3 from Quatrano N, Stevenson M, Sclafani A, et al. V-Y Advancement Flap for Defects of the Lid-Cheek Junction. Facial Plastic Surgery. 2017; 33(03):329-333.

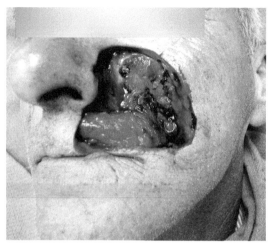

A4 from Zenn M, Jones G, ed. Reconstructive Surgery: Anatomy, Technique, and Clinical Applications. 1st Edition. Thieme; 2012.

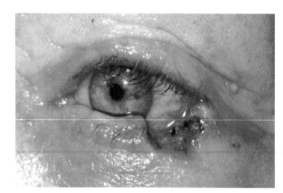

A5 from Welkoborsky H, Wiechens B, Hinni M, ed. Interdisciplinary Management of Orbital Diseases: Textbook and Atlas. 1st edition. Thieme; 2017.

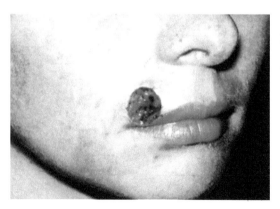

A6 from Cheney M, Hadlock T, ed. Facial Surgery: Plastic and Reconstructive. 1st Edition. Thieme; 2014.

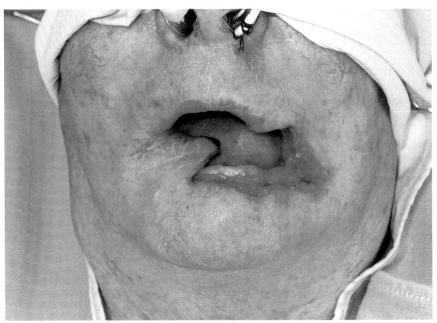

A7 from Hanasono M, Robb G, Skoracki R, et al., ed. Reconstructive Plastic Surgery of the Head and Neck: Current Techniques and Flap Atlas. 1st edition. Thieme; 2016.

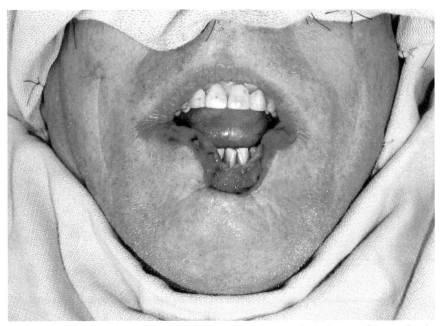

A8 from Hanasono M, Robb G, Skoracki R, et al., ed. Reconstructive Plastic Surgery of the Head and Neck: Current Techniques and Flap Atlas. 1st edition. Thieme; 2016.

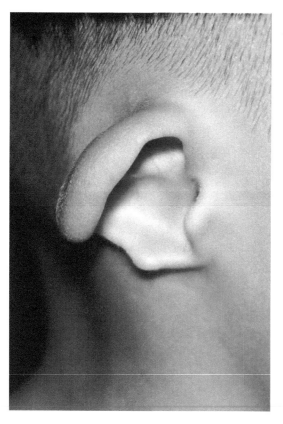

A9 from Papel I, Rodel J, Holt R, et al., ed. Facial Plastic and Reconstructive Surgery. 4th Edition. Thieme; 2016.

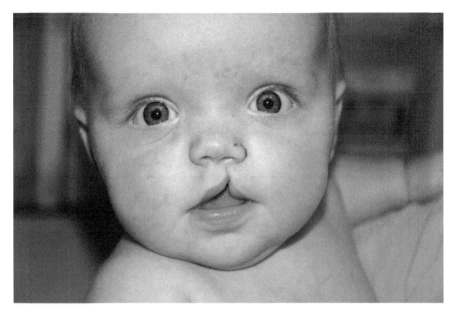

A10 from Losee J, Kirschner R, ed. Comprehensive Cleft Care. 2nd Edition. Thieme; 2015.

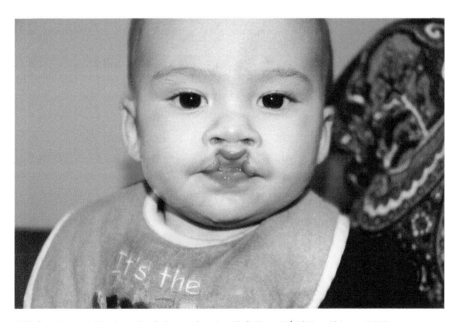

A11 from Losee J, Kirschner R, ed. Comprehensive Cleft Care. 2nd Edition. Thieme; 2015.

Appendix B: Suggested Reconstructions

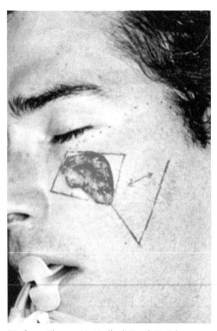

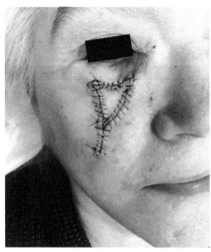

B2 from Quatrano N, Stevenson M, Sclafani A, et al. V-Y Advancement Flap for Defects of the Lid-Cheek Junction. Facial Plastic Surgery. 2017; 33(03):329-333.

B1 from Cheney M, Hadlock T, ed. Facial Surgery: Plastic and Reconstructive. 1st Edition. Thieme; 2014.

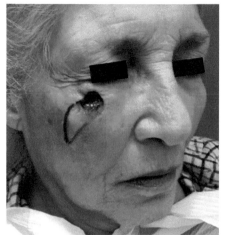
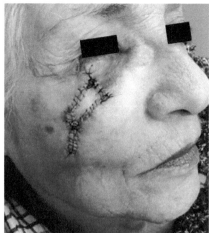

B3 from Quatrano N, Stevenson M, Sclafani A, et al. V-Y Advancement Flap for Defects of the Lid-Cheek Junction. Facial Plastic Surgery. 2017; 33(03):329-333.

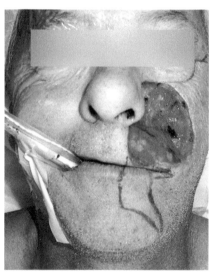

B4 from Zenn M, Jones G, ed. Reconstructive Surgery: Anatomy, Technique, and Clinical Applications. 1st Edition. Thieme; 2012.

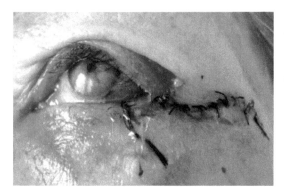

B5 from Welkoborsky H, Wiechens B, Hinni M, ed. Interdisciplinary Management of Orbital Diseases: Textbook and Atlas. 1st edition. Thieme; 2017.

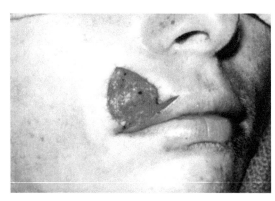

B6 from Cheney M, Hadlock T, ed. Facial Surgery: Plastic and Reconstructive. 1st Edition. Thieme; 2014.

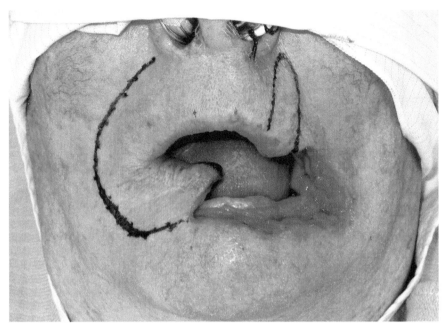

B7 from Hanasono M, Robb G, Skoracki R, et al., ed. Reconstructive Plastic Surgery of the Head and Neck: Current Techniques and Flap Atlas. 1st edition. Thieme; 2016.

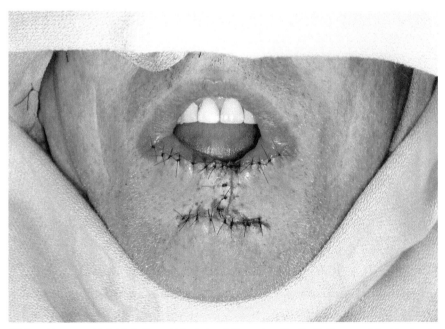

B8 from Hanasono M, Robb G, Skoracki R, et al., ed. Reconstructive Plastic Surgery of the Head and Neck: Current Techniques and Flap Atlas. 1st edition. Thieme; 2016.

Index

Note: Page numbers followed by *f* and *t* indicate figures and tables, respectively.